*Comments on Eczema – the 'at y...
from readers*

'I think the book is very good and answers the questions in a simple and easy to understand way.'

Sue Ward, Information and Education Manager,
National Eczema Society

'I learnt a lot even though I have had bad eczema for several years. I particularly liked the chapters dealing with the psychological aspects of this disease – I wish this had been available 10 years ago.'

Lesley Cumming, Tonbridge

AT YOUR FINGERTIPS

ECZEMA

Dr Tim Mitchell MRGCP, DRCOG, DPD
General Practitioner, Montpelier Health Centre;
Adviser to the All Party Parliamentary Group on Skin;
Founder Member of the Primary Care Dermatology Society

Alison Hepplewhite BSc (Hons), RGN, ENB 264, N25
Dermatology Nurse Specialist,
Bristol North Primary Health Care Trust

 6/2037530

CLASS PUBLISHING • LONDON

Printing history
First published 2006

The authors and publishers welcome feedback from the users of this book. Please contact the publishers.

Class Publishing (London) Ltd,
Barb House, Barb Mews, London W6 7PA
Telephone: 020 7371 2119
Fax: 020 7371 2878 [International +4420]
Email: post@class.co.uk
www.class.co.uk

The information presented in this book is accurate and current to the best of the authors' knowledge. The authors and publisher, however, make no guarantee as to, and assume no responsibility for, the correctness, sufficiency or completeness of such information or recommendation. The reader is advised to consult a doctor regarding all aspects of individual health care.

A CIP catalogue record for this book is available from the British Library

ISBN 10: 1859591256

ISBN 13: 9781859591253

Edited by Carrie Walker

Cartoons by Jane Taylor

Typeset by Martin Bristow

Printed and bound in Finland by WS Bookwell, Juva

Contents

Acknowledgements

We are grateful to all the people who have helped in the production of this book, and in particular we thank the following for their contributions and support:

- all those with eczema who provided the questions

- Sue Ward, Information and Education Manager, National Eczema Society for providing questions and checking the manuscript

- the National Eczema Society, whose staff are always willing to help.

Foreword

by Margaret Cox

Chief Executive, National Eczema Society

If you have eczema, you can be sure that everyone else will know a 'cure'. It is all too easy to be overwhelmed by conflicting and sometimes inaccurate advice, as well as to underestimate the impact of eczema physically and on a person's social and family life. What a joy therefore to have a new book which is medically accurate, wide ranging and practical in its approach.

Eczema is a highly individual condition. Those of us who live with it may over time come to realise that what works for one person does not necessarily work for another. Although there are many common trigger factors, not all of them will necessarily affect each of us. But identifying these be a long, frustrating and sometimes miserable process.

By addressing the issues that people with eczema, parents and carers most commonly want information about in a straightforward question-and-answer format, this new guide offers valuable advice and loads of useful hints and tips to help them to take control of the condition.

There is as yet no cure for eczema, but if it can be managed, the improvement to quality of life can be immense. The National Eczema Society welcomes this new guide as a very useful tool in helping people towards that goal.

THE CHARTER
FOR PEOPLE WITH ECZEMA

In common with all patients, people with eczema need:

- Respect for their well-being, dignity, individual needs and privacy; also for their personal wishes concerning the relief of pain or termination of treatment.

- Safety through adequate staffing, well-maintained premises and equipment, proper investment in training and research, and thorough vetting of new drugs and medical procedures.

- Redress when things go wrong which is timely and appropriate and includes courteous explanations and apologies where necessary.

In particular, people with eczema need:

- Access to the full range of services when and where they are needed. Difficulties with language, costs, mobility or the long-term nature of eczema should not be a barrier to care.

- Full diagnosis and explanation of the type of eczema and its possible causes. Prognosis, including information on the possible impact on life-style, and demonstration and instructions on the appropriate use of medications and treatments, such as bandages.

- Respect for and recognition of the intellectual capacity, experience and knowledge of the patient and representative or carer. The nature and volatility of eczema are such that their observations should be fully taken into account by the medical team and used when decisions are made on improving and monitoring health care.

- Assurance of adequate primary health care resources to enable routine treatment to be conducted in the community rather than in hospital. The good of the patient should be considered a priority against costs in areas such as:
  - receiving adequate supplies of medications, dressings and aids;
  - adequate training for the primary health care team in teaching about the appropriate use of medications or bandages.

- The right of choice to change GPs, have a second opinion, be consulted on treatment, hospital care or sex of doctor, or the freedom to use complementary medicine, all without prejudice to continued support. The nature and state of knowledge and the multifactorial nature of eczema mean that a range of treatments and a policy of caring for and understanding of the whole person are important.

- Communication by health professionals in clear and comprehensible terms and adequate to the patient's needs. This could include options for treatment, clinical trials, likely outcomes, waiting times, complaints procedures and offer of access to the NES, its information, publications and support systems.

- Guidance on general or specific requirements in relation to life-style, education, employment and welfare benefits, recognising that ignorance about eczema in the community can result in misunderstanding, stigma and discrimination. Use of NES literature can help patients reach their full potential.

- Consistency, continuity and accountability of medical care through a clearly defined chain of command so that there is always a specified person or department who is responsible for an individual's care. The many causes of eczema and aspects of treatment make this of particular importance.

- Immediacy of consultation, recognising that eczema can flare to acute proportions in a matter of hours. The 'open appointment' system should be made available to all identified as needing this service.

- Communication between systems of medical care where a patient needs treatment from other specialties; e.g. when a person with eczema requires treatment for asthma or is in a surgical ward, or when a child with eczema is cared for in a paediatric ward.

- Confidentiality of medical records and entitlement of private examination if requested, recognising that eczema can be a disfiguring and potentially embarrassing condition.

- Continuing support, especially if the eczema becomes chronic and palliative care is required, together with care and support over periods of acute ill-health caused by the eczema.

- Consideration of family needs and the particularly disruptive nature of eczema, which can affect partners, carers and siblings. Their particular needs should be recognized as linked but separate from those of the person with eczema.

Introduction

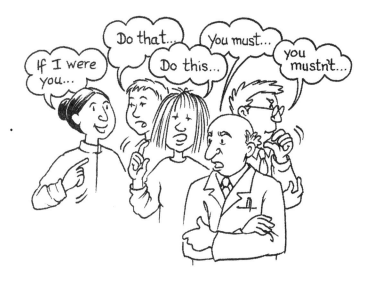

Most people probably do not think of the skin as anything other than our outer layer, but it is really an organ. Just like the liver or the kidneys, it carries out several different and important functions, and although it seems very thin, it is in fact the largest organ in the body. It has a surface area of 1.8 m^2 and makes up about 16% of body weight. Before looking at the causes and impact of a skin disease such as eczema, it is worth listing the more important functions of the skin:

- a barrier to physical agents including ultraviolet radiation;

- protection against mechanical injury;

- a defence against microbes;

- homeostasis – preventing the loss of water and electrolytes;

- a temperature regulator and insulator;

- sensory functions;

- fine touch and grip;

- vitamin D synthesis;

- a calorie store – in the subcutaneous fat;

- cosmetic, psychosocial and display functions.

Any disease that has an effect on even a few of these functions is likely to have an effect on the functioning of the whole person, both physically and psychologically. Eczema is one of these diseases and can have a variety of different causes and names. Atopic eczema is probably the best known, but there are also contact eczema, which can be irritant or allergic, discoid eczema, seborrhoeic eczema and eczema associated with poor circulation in the legs and varicose veins – referred to as venous, varicose, stasis or gravitational eczema.

Atopic eczema is the most common chronic skin disease in childhood, and although the majority of cases clear up before adulthood, the affected person remains vulnerable to recurrences. Cases that persist, and these recurrences, seem to have an important element of irritation from, or allergy to, a variety of substances that come into contact with the skin. Contact eczema is much more important to consider with eczema in adults than in children. This book may seem to concentrate on atopic eczema but, as it is the main type, much of the research into eczema and its treatments are based on this, and the basic problem in the skin is much the same for the different types. As will be shown later, the principles of treatment are also similar.

Eczema is a very common problem. In the UK, skin problems account for somewhere between 15% and 20% of all consultations in general practice, and eczema accounts for 30% of these – 5% of all patients seeing a GP. In hospital dermatology departments, where many of the less common conditions are concentrated, eczema accounts for 14% of the work.

As previously mentioned, the effects of eczema are not just physical – it has a psychological effect as well. One recent survey of the effects of eczema on quality of life came up with the following findings:

- 33% said that eczema had impacted on their work/school, home and social life;

- 14% said that their career progression had been affected by eczema, whether through limiting their choice of career or through poor performance at interview;

- 36% found that flares affected their self-confidence;

- 51% felt unhappy or depressed during flares;

- 21% admitted to difficulty in forming relationships;

- 41% of those in established relationships said that they felt awkward about partners seeing or touching their bodies;

- 30% of patients and carers said that eczema had an impact on the lives of other members of the household;

- only 26% said that their doctor had discussed the emotional impact of eczema with them.

It is so important for people with eczema to feel able to discuss the emotional aspects of their skin problems – we hope this book helps them to demand some help and support.

The more physical aspects of treating eczema can also raise problems. Deciding what is best for your skin can be very difficult and is not helped by conflicting advice from different sources. One patient said that he felt more people had an opinion about eczema than about who should be picked for the England football team! For example:

- the neighbour says, 'You shouldn't have a bath more than once a week';

- the nurse says, 'You should have a bath every day';

- the GP says, 'Weak topical steroids are safe';

- the pharmacist says, 'They cause skin thinning';

- the specialist says, 'Use this steroid on the face';

- the packaging on the steroid says, 'Do not use on the face'.

The information provided by the manufacturer can also say 'Do not use on broken skin' and/or 'Use sparingly'. It's very easy to get confused! You feel that all eczema looks like 'broken skin', and what does 'sparingly' mean? You may well ask why there are so many seemingly contradictory opinions about this skin disorder, and there may be a number of explanations:

- There is no single correct treatment for eczema. Many different treatment approaches may produce the same outcome, and all may be equally worthwhile. Wherever possible, therapy should be tailored to the wishes of each individual.

- What works for one person may not work for another.

- The most important aspect of eczema treatment relies on the application of creams or ointments to the skin yet scant regard is paid to instructions on how to apply these, how frequently and in what quantities. If these issues are not adequately explained or demonstrated, treatment will not be used correctly, leading to apparent 'treatment failure' even when the therapy is appropriate.

- The natural history of eczema is that it will get better and worsen again regardless of therapy. This can be through the avoidance of certain triggers, but in most instances we cannot explain why this happens. It is only natural to look at anything that has happened before any such change (e.g. a different diet, a new herbal remedy, a change in the weather) and see this as the cause. Unfortunately, this can lead to false hope of having found a 'cure' – and inevitable disappointment.

- We are sorry to say that the lack of dermatology training among people in the medical and allied professions does not help to improve their understanding of the problems caused by eczema and other skin diseases. Many of the people who contributed questions to this book were unhappy about the treatment given by their GP and about the general lack of empathy and support. This is a common complaint, and doctors' training needs to be changed before the situation will dramatically improve. Eczema can make up 5% of a GP's workload, yet it is possible to become a GP without any formal training in dealing with skin disease. A great many GPs are very good at treating eczema, but this is usually because they have recognised the need to take the time, trouble and often expense to learn a lot more about it.

- There can even be some confusion over the difference between the words 'eczema' and 'dermatitis'. Eczema comes from a Greek word for 'boiling' – a good description of how the skin can feel in acute eczema. Dermatitis really means 'inflammation of the skin' so could be used for other forms of disease that cause inflammation. The word 'dermatitis' was often taken to mean that the skin problem was caused by an external factor and, if the person was in work, some form of compensation might be involved. Some forms of eczema are often referred to as dermatitis – the seborrhoeic form and when the napkin area is affected – but it is better to stick to using 'eczema' to avoid confusion.

In *Eczema – the 'at your fingertips' guide*, we hope to lead you through the maze of fact and fiction concerning eczema, its causes and its management. We freely acknowledge that we do not have all the answers, but we will try to provide a sensible approach based on our experience of dealing with the many different types of eczema. We do not claim that ours is the only valid approach, but we hope that it will prove educational and of practical use in your day-to-day management of this common skin disorder.

1
What is eczema?

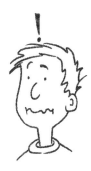

Introduction

The term 'eczema' is used for a group of conditions that show a similar pattern of changes in the skin, giving rise to specific changes on the surface. The word itself comes from the Greek and means 'to boil or flow out' – anyone who has had acute eczema will understand how appropriate this is.

In acute (short-term) eczema, intense inflammation leads to the formation of little blisters (vesicles) in the skin, which soon burst or are scratched open, leading to weeping and the 'flowing out' of fluid. Even if there are no vesicles, a section of skin affected by eczema looked at under a microscope shows fluid between the skin cells, tending to push them apart. This produces an appearance reminiscent of a sponge – hence the term 'spongiosis' that is used by doctors. All the different conditions called eczema would be expected to show this spongiosis, together with some degree of inflammation around superficial blood vessels, which are dilated, producing the hot, red feeling and appearance.

7

Is there a simple way of classifying eczema?

Unfortunately, no.

There are many different causes and triggers for eczema – some from the outside world, for example irritants, allergy and bacterial infection, and others from within the body. The ones from within are called 'intrinsic' and include 'atopy' – having a genetic tendency to eczema, asthma and hay fever – raised pressure in the leg veins, and reactions to stressful circumstances. These causes and trigger factors are not mutually exclusive, so several may be important at the same time in the same person; it is, however, usually possible to give a general label to the main underlying cause.

As well as trying to provide an appropriate label, it is often useful to classify eczema in terms of how long it has been there and how quickly it appeared. Calling it 'acute' suggests a rapid onset and a short but maybe severe course; 'chronic' means continuing for a long time. This time course may give some extra clues to the trigger or triggers involved.

Most classifications are imperfect but do serve to show the different factors involved in producing similar changes in the skin.

Eczema can be classified as follows:

1. *Mainly caused by external triggers.*

- Irritant – various chemicals, including detergents in soap.
- Physical factors – friction and chronic rubbing, sunlight and artificial ultraviolet light.
- Allergic – the immune system reacting to something coming into contact with the skin or taken by mouth.

2. *Internal and other causes.*

- Atopic – often associated with hay fever, asthma and food allergies.
- Seborrhoeic – related to yeasts on the skin, which has a specific pattern.
- Discoid – a descriptive term for rounded patches of eczema with no obvious cause.

- Venous/varicose/gravitational/stasis – a number of different terms for eczema on the lower legs owing to problems with the blood flow and pressure in the superficial veins, which can be varicose.

- Asteatotic – usually in elderly people and caused by excessive washing and dry, low-humidity environments. The skin takes on an appearance like crazy paving.

- Pompholyx – lots of very itchy blisters on the hands and feet.

- Neuro-dermatitis – often called lichen simplex, this is linked to chronic rubbing or scratching.

Is eczema the same as dermatitis?

Yes, and no!

'Dermatitis' is a more generalised word, simply meaning inflammation of the skin. All eczema is dermatitis, but many other conditions that can be called dermatitis fall within the grouping of dermatitis. Most of the different types of eczema can, and often are, interchangeably termed dermatitis – the term is more commonly used in the USA. Previously more than now, an eczematous process caused by an irritant or allergic problem in the workplace was called contact dermatitis, and issues concerning compensation might at least have been implied.

For some types of eczema, it is more commonplace to use 'dermatitis'. Cases include napkin (diaper) dermatitis, photo-dermatitis and neuro-dermatitis. For others, for example asteatotic eczema, 'eczema' has been the preferred term. For some of the rest – such as seborrhoeic and discoid – eczema and dermatitis are used interchangeably. The situation is therefore still very confusing, and it is always worth asking your doctor if he or she means something different from your understanding of the words.

What is atopic eczema?

This comes from the word 'atopy', which refers to a group of conditions in which the immune system reacts to allergens in the environment by producing raised levels of immunoglobulin type E (IgE), which in turn leads to the changes in the skin. Seventy-five per cent of cases present before the age of 6 months, rising to 90% before the age of 5 years. It is thought to affect 3% of infants and persists for several years. Of the children affected, 60–70% will have gone into remission (no longer suffer from eczema) by their early teenage years, although they remain vulnerable to recurrences and may always have problems with dry skin. The pattern of rash on the skin varies with age:

- In infancy, it often starts on the face with vesicles and weeping. Distribution elsewhere is non-specific, but it does tend to spare the napkin area.

- As the child ages, the distribution becomes more flexural around knees, elbows, wrists and ankles. The skin becomes increasingly thickened, dry and excoriated – often looking 'leathery' (lichenification).

This pattern continues into adulthood, with increasing lichenification and an increasing tendency to affect the trunk, face and hands.

Will I ever grow out of my atopic eczema? I am now in my thirties!

Unfortunately, most adults who have atopic eczema that has persisted from childhood tend to find that it continues into old age. It is therefore very important that you work hard on finding a treatment regime that allows you to manage it as easily as possible.

The health visitor says that my baby has cradle cap and that this is a type of eczema. Is this true?

Yes, this is a type of eczema called seborrhoeic eczema. It may affect infants but is rare during later childhood. It is probably most common in men. It has several different patterns but most commonly affects the face and scalp in infants as well as the napkin area. Unlike atopic eczema, it does not feel itchy, so your baby won't scratch very much. There are three main patterns:

- A red, scaly rash on the scalp and ears, around the nose and in the creases down to the lips and eyebrows. It is often associated with eczema in the ear canals and on the eyelids. This is the 'cradle cap' your health visitor is referring to.

- On the trunk in the centre of the chest and upper back. There is a dry, scaly rash sometimes accompanied by a more extensive outbreak of little bumps and spots around the hair follicles.

- An intertriginous form affecting the armpits, belly button and groins, which can also present under spectacles or hearing aids.

My baby has bad nappy rash despite regular changing and the use of a barrier cream. Could she have a form of eczema?

There are actually three types of eczema that can affect the nappy area. The most common is irritant eczema (nappy rash), which can affect nearly all babies to some extent. This simply reflects the fact that urine and faeces are irritant to the skin if left in contact with it for prolonged periods. This type of nappy rash usually spares the skin right in the groins. The skin fold between the leg and the tummy therefore looks normal but is surrounded on either side by red, inflamed skin.

As you are already doing all the right things to prevent nappy rash, your baby may have one of the other types of eczema (atopic or seborrhoeic). Both of these tend to involve rather than spare the skin fold at the top of the leg. Atopic eczema only rarely affects the nappy area and is normally very itchy. You may see eczema in the skin folds elsewhere on the body (e.g. in front of the elbows or behind the knees). In contrast, seborrhoeic eczema tends not to be itchy and tends to be associated with greasy yellow scales on the scalp (cradle cap).

I am 45 and have never had any problems with my skin. I now have itchy, round, scaly patches on my arms and legs that my GP says are eczema. Is this right?

Yes, these could be, although your GP may also have considered other causes such as fungal infection and psoriasis. This pattern is called discoid eczema. The precise cause of this has yet to be identified, but chronic stress and local infection may play a part.

As you have found, the rash typically presents on the limbs in people in their forties and fifties, and it is more common in men. Unlike atopic eczema, it favours the extensor surfaces and appears as round 'plaques' rather than being more spread out. These plaques are usually 5 cm or less in diameter. Looking closely at them, you should see some tiny little blisters and crusting where the fluid from the blisters has dried. The underlying skin will probably be thickened. Discoid eczema can be very stubborn and difficult to treat, so it may persist for many months.

I had eczema as a child, but it cleared up until recently when I got it again on my hands. Why is this?

It sounds as though you have a form of eczema caused by contact with irritant chemicals. Not surprisingly, this is called 'irritant contact eczema', and it is the most common form caused by contact (perhaps 80% of cases), the other cause being allergic. Strong irritants will cause an obvious and acute reaction on anybody's skin, but weaker irritants need months or years of exposure to cause the same problems. As you have found, the eczema usually affects the hands and forearms as the most common parts of the body exposed to detergents, industrial oils, solvents, etc. Many people with dry or fair skin are likely to develop irritant problems, but your history of atopic eczema doubles the risk.

Is hand eczema different from other eczemas?

As far as the basic underlying process in the skin goes, it is the same as other types of eczema. It can be caused by a variety of different types of eczema, so the common thing is the site – on the hands. A background of atopic eczema, wet work and contact seems to be the most important factor, and it affects women more than men. Environmental triggers from wet work and contact seem to be more important than any genetic factors. It can be a very long-lasting form of eczema, especially if it starts at a young age and is not caused by any specific allergies. It has been estimated to affect more than 1% of the adult population in the UK.

My son has what looks like eczema but just round his mouth. What might have caused it?

This could be another form of irritant eczema. If it looks red and dry with cracks or fissures, it is probably 'lip-licking' eczema. It might also be linked to irritation from, or even allergy to, toothpaste.

I get eczema under my watch strap but nowhere else. Is it some sort of allergy?

If the watch strap is metal, you could be allergic to nickel and have allergic contact eczema. This is different from irritant contact eczema in several ways as it is a type of immune problem called a delayed hypersensitivity reaction. The key points about it are:

- previous contact is necessary to induce the response;
- the response is specific to one substance;
- all areas of skin will react once sensitisation has taken place;
- sensitisation persists indefinitely, and desensitisation is unlikely to be possible.

Various patterns are seen, depending on the original site of contact. Your case is typical of nickel allergy, which can also be seen under jewellery and metal fastenings in clothing, such as the studs in jeans. Other patterns include fingertip eczema from garlic, and eczema on the face and neck from perfume. An allergic cause should be suspected if the pattern of eczema is unusual – eyelids, around leg ulcers, hands or feet – if there is a known exposure to some of the common allergens, or if the type of work is 'high risk', for example hairdressing, nursing, gardening or floristry.

My gran has very itchy legs with not much to see other than dry skin with a sort of criss-cross pattern. She used to get eczema as a child but says it didn't look like this.

She probably has asteatotic eczema, which occurs in older people who may have had eczema in the past or have, at least, a tendency to have dry skin. It is made worse by low humidity in centrally heated rooms and the removal of the natural oils from washing with soap. Diuretics can increase the problem from dehydration, and hypothyroidism should be excluded. As with your gran, it presents on the legs, which itch and show a background of dry skin with a superficial network of fine red lines giving a 'crazy paving' appearance. These fines lines are actually small cracks or fissures in the skin. Treatment with water tablets (diuretics), for blood pressure or heart problems, can make it worse, as can having a thyroid gland that is not working very well.

My doctor says that my varicose veins have caused eczema. Is he right?

Yes, it sounds as though you have venous eczema, also called varicose, stasis or gravitational eczema. It is linked to poor blood flow in the veins in the lower legs, sometimes after clots in the deep veins. The eczema is chronic, and the legs can become stained a browny colour from blood pigments getting into the skin. You will have to be very careful not to scratch the skin as it will be very fragile and prone to ulceration. If this does happen, you will need dressings and bandages; these can sometimes, however, lead to extra problems of allergic contact eczema, so be careful and look after your skin.

I have suffered from eczema since I was a child. In my adult years it has changed, and my GP has told me it was something called 'pomphlics'. What is this?

'Pompholyx' is a word used to describe a pattern of eczema affecting the hands and feet that typically shows blistering and is very itchy. There are recurring outbreaks of tense, thick-walled vesicles or larger blisters on the palms, along the fingers and sometimes on the soles of the feet. Each outbreak can last a few weeks and recur at irregular intervals. It is more common in hot weather and can occur in three types:

- in association with atopic eczema;

- linked to allergic contact eczema – people allergic to nickel may also develop it in response to low levels of nickel in food;

- in isolation (the cause here being unknown).

Are some types of eczema more common at different ages?

The age of onset can be helpful in deciding what type(s) of eczema a person has. Eczema in an infant is most commonly atopic (although this may appear discoid in places and can be aggravated by irritants) or seborrhoeic. In the child and teenager, atopic eczema is most common, but there will be some instances of contact allergy, for example to nickel. In adults of working age, irritant, contact allergic, seborrhoeic, discoid and atopic eczema are all common and can occur at many body sites; pompholyx and venous eczema are recognisable by their locations. The elderly are prone to asteatotic eczema, especially on the shins, in addition to the types experienced by younger adults.

Does it look the same in the acute and chronic stages?

Acute eczema will occur quite quickly – hours or a few days – sometimes in previously normal skin. Little blisters may appear and then break to give a weeping surface. The underlying skin will be red, perhaps swollen and often a little bumpy. Most acute eczema is very itchy, but when the skin surface has broken down, this may be replaced by soreness. As days go by, crusting and then scaling may occur alongside the weeping or gradually replace it.

'Chronic eczema' is eczema that has been present for a long time – usually at least weeks. The ongoing inflammation, rubbing and scratching all contribute to an increased thickness of the skin, which may develop a leathery appearance and show much more prominent skin surface markings. In dark skin, there may be changes in the pigmentation – both an increase and a decrease are possible. This thickened skin is liable to split, producing painful fissures, especially over the joints.

I get very confused by all the different types of eczema that can affect the skin. You say that the final process in the skin is the same for all of them. Why can't we just call it eczema and get on with treating it?

Despite the fact that, at microscopic level, the skin looks very similar in the different types of eczema, this is the end stage as the skin can only behave in so many different ways when disordered. The main reason for trying to label the different patterns accurately is that the cause, severity and outcome vary enormously between the different eczemas. Whereas some of the treatments are similar for the different types, there are many that are more specific, so accurate diagnosis is essential. Treating eczema is also not just about creams: it must involve prevention, and this is much more possible in some types than in others.

What happens in the skin?

What happens in the skin of people with eczema?

To explain what happens in eczema, you need to understand the structure of the skin as seen down a microscope. The skin consists of three layers:

- The outer layer is called the *epidermis*. This contains a 'brick wall' of skin cells (keratinocytes) that are held together by a cement (the mortar) mostly made up of fats or lipids. The many different layers start with live cells that constantly reproduce, creating new cells that move up to the surface, die and are shed. This whole process takes about 28 days. The lipid cement makes the brick wall into a very effective barrier against the environment. It prevents the skin losing too much water and prevents noxious (poisonous) substances getting in.

- The middle layer is called the *dermis*. This consists of tough structural fibres called collagen and elastin, which provide strength and elasticity to the skin. It also contains blood vessels that supply nutrients and oxygen to both the dermis and the epidermis.

- The deepest layer of the skin is called the *subcutis* and is predominantly made up of an insulating layer of fat.

In eczema, it is the dermis and epidermis that are affected. The epidermis shows the most marked changes. The inflammation leads to leaky blood vessels, so fluid collects between the keratinocytes, causing them to separate. The brick wall takes on a sponge-like appearance. As the eczema becomes chronic, the constant rubbing and scratching causes the epidermis to regenerate more quickly, so it becomes thickened.

Finally, eczema causes changes in the upper part of the dermis. This region becomes flooded with white blood cells, which are part of the body's immune system or defences. They leak out of vessels and even pass up into the epidermis. Current evidence suggests that it is these cells that drive the whole process of inflammation in the skin.

Is the skin just a simple barrier?

No, it is much more than that, and this accounts for the many physical and psychological effects that it can have, especially if you are badly affected by eczema. It is the last line of defence against the outside world, protecting our bodies from external attack and keeping the right conditions inside (homeostasis) through its prevention of loss of fluid and regulation of temperature. It also allows for a display of individuality through decoration, jewellery and hair-styling.

Skin, therefore:

- acts as a barrier to physical agents including ultraviolet radiation;
- protects against mechanical injury;
- defends against microbes;
- is involved in homeostasis – preventing the loss of water and electrolytes;
- regulates temperature and insulates;
- is involved in sensory functions;
- is integral to fine touch and grip;
- is the site of vitamin D synthesis;
- acts as a calorie store in the subcutaneous fat;
- has cosmetic, psychosocial and display functions.

Why does my skin weep fluid and feel wet?

If you think of the epidermis changing to look like a sponge, you can imagine the fluid leaking out and making the outer layer stretch up into blisters. Once these break, you will be left with a wet weeping area as the skin has lost its barrier function.

Why is skin with eczema so susceptible to irritants?

As fluid accumulates in the epidermis, the 'bricks' separate and the 'cement' becomes disrupted, leaving big cracks in the 'barrier'. Irritants that would normally be kept on the surface are allowed through to the more sensitive dermis. Some irritants, such as soaps, act to dissolve the lipid-based cement, leading to a further breakdown of the skin's barrier function.

How does our doctor know that my child's rash is eczema?

As there are no specific tests for most types of eczema, your doctor will have reached a diagnosis on what we call 'clinical grounds'. This means taking a careful history of the problem and any family history of eczema, asthma or hay fever. Examination of the skin will add to the clues in the history, allowing a diagnosis to be made.

Some people with atopic eczema may have abnormal blood tests, such as high levels of an antibody called immunoglobulin E (IgE). Antibodies are chemicals made by the body as a defence against infection but are also involved in allergic reactions. Specific allergens (the causes or triggers of allergy) can lead to high levels of linked IgE, which can be measured by a blood test called an ELISA test. (This is discussed in Chapter 2 under allergy testing.) These tests do not, however, diagnose atopic eczema as you can have abnormal tests and never develop eczema, or have normal IgE levels and very definite eczema.

My family are from India and I have noticed that my eczema looks different from eczema in my friends with white skin. Why is this?

I am afraid that we cannot explain why there are different patterns of eczema in different racial groups, but you are right to have spotted the difference. Eczema often affects the flexures (the creases in front of the elbows and behind the knees), but in Asian and particularly in African/Caribbean people, eczema sometimes shows a reverse pattern, affecting the extensor surfaces (behind the elbows and the front of the knees). There can be other differences in the way in which pigmented skin reacts giving rise to unusual presentations of eczema:

- Thickening of the skin (lichenification) seems to happen much more readily.

- Lumps or papules are more common, giving a raised, bumpy appearance to the skin.

- There may be a marked increase or decrease in pigmentation of the skin after the eczema has settled down. This can be very distressing as it can be quite disfiguring.

Why does it itch?

Why does skin itch with eczema?

Surprisingly, this is a very difficult question to answer as the current scientific understanding of itch is really very poor. We do know that certain small nerve fibres in the skin transmit 'itch' signals to the spinal cord and then to the brain. These same fibres can also transmit pain signals. There are certain centres in the brain that receive these signals and then interpret them either as an itch sensation or sometimes as pain. Two different types of nerve fibre are involved, one being faster than the other. This explains why itching can be made up of an early localised pricking sensation followed by a diffuse itching or burning sensation.

Why people with eczema itch isn't really known, but it may be that the dry, inflamed skin of eczema fires off these nerve fibres, causing the itch. There is, however, also some evidence that these nerve fibres and the chemical signals (neurotransmitters) that they contain may be abnormal in eczema. This could mean that the abnormal itching sensation is the first problem, with the other skin changes being 'secondary' – i.e. being the result of the damage caused by scratching. A lot more research needs to be done into the mechanisms of itch before we have a clearer picture.

Facts and figures

How many people are affected by eczema?

It is very difficult to answer this precisely as there are so many different types of eczema. Skin disease in general can make up around 15% of the workload of a GP, and a third of this is down to eczema. We know most about children with atopic eczema, and different studies suggest that as many as 15% of those living in developed countries will suffer from eczema at some time. This percentage has been gradually increasing over the past 30 years.

Do boys get eczema more than girls?

Yes, atopic eczema is a little more common in boys than girls.

When does eczema start?

It depends what sort of eczema you are talking about. The most common form, atopic eczema, starts in childhood, and the earlier it starts, the more likely the child is to grow out of it. For example, if it starts before the age of 1, there is a more than 90% chance of growing out of it before adult life. Contact eczema, often affecting the hands, tends to come on in adult life, especially if there is a history of atopic eczema. About 5–10% of children with atopic eczema will develop hand eczema in adult life even if they have grown out of their original eczema. This is especially true if they take up certain careers (e.g. as a hairdresser, mechanic or nurse) that lead to repeated irritation and damage to the hands.

Do people with eczema have a higher chance of developing asthma?

Atopic eczema, asthma and hay fever tend to go together as 'atopic' diseases. Asthma is a common disease in its own right as it affects up to 10% of people at some time in their life. A child with eczema has an increased risk of suffering from asthma as well – perhaps

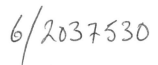
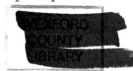

up to a 50% chance. Eczema tends to start earlier in life, and research is being done to see whether any form of treatment for the eczema will make later asthma less likely.

I moved to England from Jamaica 16 years ago. Two of my children have eczema, and I have other friends who also have affected children. Is eczema more common in the UK than in the West Indies?

Yes, it seems that eczema is much more common in the UK. One recent study showed that eczema is almost twice as common among schoolchildren in London than in Kingston, Jamaica. When just the black children were studied, the difference was even more marked – eczema was up to four times more common in London. This difference also seems to apply to Indian and Bangladeshi populations living in the UK.

What if it isn't eczema?

For several years, I have been getting recurrent crops of dry yellow blisters that come up on my hands on the palm side. They seem to start deep in the skin and end up on the surface as a brown scale. Is this a form of eczema?

This sounds as though it is a condition called palmar pustulosis, which can also affect the soles of the feet, when it is called palmo-plantar pustulosis. The yellow blisters you describe contain pus that is sterile, so not caused by an infection. Pus is just a collection of white cells, which are involved in inflammation as well as fighting infection. As they come up to the surface, the pustules dry up so that only a dry discoloured patch of skin is left. This condition is thought to have features of both eczema and another skin problem called psoriasis and can be quite difficult to treat.

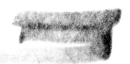

What is the difference between eczema and psoriasis?

They are both capable of producing widespread chronic rashes, but psoriasis is a disease in which the turnover of the skin is greatly speeded up – from the normal of 28 days down to 3 or 4. It therefore produces much more scale than eczema and the rash is much more 'demarcated', so you can see when it stops and normal skin takes over. It can be confused with eczema on certain parts of the body such as the face, hands and feet, and with certain types of eczema such as discoid eczema, in which there also tends to be scaling and discrete patches. Psoriasis involves parts of the immune system in the skin that are different from the ones involved in eczema, so it is rare to have both diseases together.

Are there any other diseases that are less common if you have eczema?

High blood pressure (hypertension) seems to be rare in adults with atopic eczema, whether it is active or not. This has been found in studies, but no definite reason has yet been established.

When I saw a dermatologist about my eczema, he said I also had keratosis pilaris and gave me a cream for that – I thought it was all part of my eczema, but have I got two diseases?

Keratosis pilaris is a common condition in which the hair follicles in the skin become filled with plugs of keratin. It usually begins in childhood and tends to improve as you get older. The outer aspects of the upper arms and thighs feel rough because of the plugging of the follicles and can look red. Many people have a very mild form of it, but it does seem to be more common in people with atopic eczema. You do have another disease but one that is associated with having eczema. Creams that help to soften and 'dissolve' the keratin plugs are known as 'keratolytics', and this may be what the doctor has given you. They will only ever have a temporary effect on the skin, so you need to keep using them.

My husband is 51 and has redness and itching on his eyelids, spreading to his cheeks. Is this eczema?

It is very difficult to tell you what this is without more information. At his age, it could be a condition called rosacea, which can cause a red, sometimes bumpy, rash over the cheeks that can be associated with irritation of the eyelids – called blepharitis. Rosacea can also cause flushing and a burning feeling in the face after alcohol, spicy foods or a sudden change of temperature. He should see his GP as the steroid creams used to treat eczema can sometimes cause rosacea if used for too long a time.

These days I only have mild eczema, but I recently developed blister eczema in the middle of the sole of one foot. It doesn't seem to respond to my usual creams and seems to be getting bigger. Is it just more stubborn than my normal eczema?

You may not have 'blister eczema', which we call pompholyx, as it is just affecting one foot. Eczema tends to affect both sides of the body, so you should be suspicious that an outbreak like this is caused by something else. The first thing to come to mind is a fungal infection, which can be quite inflamed and can cause little blisters. You should see your GP and get some skin scrapings taken to look for fungus.

Many people treat fungal infections (also known as tinea) with steroids in the mistaken belief that the rash is eczema. The steroids will damp down the inflammation in the skin and mask the infection, allowing it to spread in the skin. They then get a much larger patch of slightly itchy skin, often with a thin red line all the way round the edge where the fungus is growing – this is called 'tinea incognito' as the typical features of a fungal infection are hidden.

2
What causes eczema?

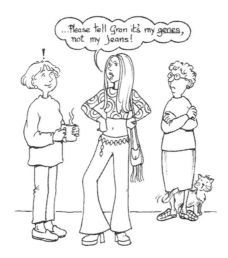

Introduction

It must be very frustrating to ask your doctor why you have eczema only to get a vague answer suggesting several possible causes. The truth is that we don't yet have a simple answer to this simple question – and we may never have. In this chapter we will try to explain what our current understanding is and, just as importantly, try to dispel some of the myths that abound. It may be easier to establish what does *not* cause eczema, but we fully understand that myths and untruths will arise if we do not fully understand the causes of eczema. It is important to do clear up misconceptions of the cause as they can lead to wholly inappropriate treatment and poorly controlled disease. If there were a simple answer to 'What causes eczema?', you would not be reading this book!

As with much of this book, we have many more answers related to studies on atopic eczema and contact eczema than on some of the other types, but the general messages are appropriate for all the different types.

Are there any common things that make eczema worse?

This depends to some extent on what type of eczema you are talking about. Much more research has been carried out in people with atopic eczema, so most of the answers to the more general questions relate more to atopic eczema than to the other forms. It is safe to say that if you have large areas of contact eczema, your skin is likely to be irritated by the same sorts of thing that have come up in studies of atopic individuals. Apart from the use of soaps and other things that can directly irritate the skin, the most common reasons are sweating (usually from exercise), fabrics (especially if the contact was at work) and hot weather. Fabrics encountered at work seem to relate not just to a direct irritant effect, but also to a physical friction effect if they have to be handled constantly as part of a job.

Inheritance and allergy

I want to find out exactly what is causing my son's eczema. How can I get him tested?

You have asked one of the most difficult questions to answer because we do not have a complete understanding of the cause or causes of the various types of eczema. Your son is likely to have atopic eczema as this is the most common childhood form, so it is unlikely to be due to a single allergy, for which avoidance of the 'allergen' (the cause or trigger of the allergy) would result in a cure. This approach might apply in contact allergic eczema, which is much more common in adult life, but even then there is usually more than one trigger.

We do know that there is a strong inherited or genetic component to atopic eczema. If you son has inherited a certain gene, or combination of genes, this predisposes him to being 'atopic', but he would still need some other trigger to cause him to have eczema. To date, several genes have been identified that show a link with atopic disease, but it seems likely that there are other, as yet unidentified, genes that are important, and we hope that these will be discovered over the next few years. We still do not understand the function of these genes as we do not know whether they can all lead to asthma, eczema or hay fever – the three atopic diseases – or whether individual genes are linked to just one of the diseases. It is more likely that various different gene combinations can lead to atopic eczema as this would help to explain why different triggers are important in different patients and why eczema has more that one 'cause'.

In other words, if your son has a susceptibility to developing eczema by having a particular group of genes, the eczema may be triggered by several different factors. Despite much research, the evidence for any one trigger is very limited, and trials excluding or limiting exposure to different environmental factors (e.g. pets, woollen clothing, dust, car pollution) have been very disappointing in terms of improving eczema. There is therefore no simple way to get your son tested, and it is more likely that simple detective work, looking at when it gets worse, may give you more of a clue. (For more about testing, though, see the section 'Are there any tests?' later in this chapter.)

But isn't eczema caused by an allergy to something?

It depends what you mean by 'allergy'. The strictly scientific definition of allergy refers to 'when a substance causes an abnormally excessive response to arise from the body's immune or defence system'. This may be measured by determining the levels of antibody in the white blood cells (lymphocytes). The allergic reaction should be reproducible by 're-challenging' with the same substance – the same reaction will be produced each time the substance is used.

Many people, however, use the word 'allergy' in a different way. They may use it to imply that a certain disorder is caused by a specific substance and that this disorder will disappear if the offending agent is avoided. Unfortunately, this is not the case with atopic eczema. It is perhaps best imagined as a built-in reaction that can be modified (but not caused) by the environment. Many things in the environment can make eczema worse (e.g. woollen clothes, dog hair), but this may be because they act purely as an irritant rather than as a true allergen.

My GP says that my hand eczema is caused by things I come in contact with. What does this really mean?

Contact is the most common cause of hand eczema in adults. Your GP's comment can be looked at in a couple of ways. First, some substances are potentially irritant to the skin such that anyone would eventually develop a rash that looked like eczema if they were exposed to high enough concentrations for long enough. An example here is strong detergent. Your problem could be that you have a much lower threshold to a wide range of possible irritants, so you react to lower concentrations and a shorter contact time. This will especially be the case if you have a little bit of eczema or just dry skin at the time of the contact. The same contact on an area of normal skin would not cause you a problem.

The other possibility is that you are allergic to a particular substance (or several if you are unlucky). This substance would be unlikely to cause any reaction in someone without an allergy to it no matter how long they were in contact with it, and it would be able to cause eczema on any part of your skin after the initial 'sensitising' reaction had taken place. Your first contact that caused a problem would lead to eczema after a few days or so, but subsequent contacts would cause the eczema to start within a matter of hours. An example of this is an allergy to something in a perfume such as 'balsam of Peru'.

What is the hygiene hypothesis?

In the late 1980s, it was noticed that large families seemed to have much less in the way of atopic disease. This was mainly found when studying asthma, for which the link is much more established than it is for atopic eczema. (The link does not apply to other types of eczema.)

It is thought that allergic diseases might be more likely to develop if the immune system of an infant or young child is understimulated from a lack of contact with infection, dirt, dust etc. The immune system is designed to allow us to develop protection against infections, so if a child is not exposed to any, the immune system finds something else to react to! No single, specific infection has been linked to atopic eczema, so this is not an argument against immunisation, but it is worth avoiding unnecessary courses of antibiotics in early life and trying to be relaxed about children playing together and sharing germs and dirt. Perhaps the old saying about 'eating a peck of dirt' has some validity. Some further support for the hypothesis has come from developing countries, where improvements in hygiene, and perhaps a better availability of treatment for worms and other gut parasites, seem to be linked to an increase in atopic disease.

What type of dog can I have that will not irritate my son's eczema?

Dogs, and indeed any animals with furry or hairy coats (e.g. horses, cats), shed their hair and skin into the environment. These small particles are made up of proteins that are 'foreign' to humans. They can irritate the skin without an allergic reaction taking place, especially if the skin is already damaged with eczema. They may also cause a genuine allergic response. Although breeds of dogs with shorter coats may spread their proteins around the house in lesser amounts, these will still be present in a significant quantity. All dogs therefore have the potential to make eczema worse, so it is probably best not to get a dog or other pet with a furry or hairy coat.

Are house dust mites involved?

What are house dust mites?

House dust mites are very small insects that are invisible to the naked eye. They are found in all of our homes, and they particularly like living in soft furnishings such as sofas, mattresses, carpets and duvets, where they are found in large numbers. Modern standards of living, with central heating, seem to encourage their growth, and in practice they are difficult to eradicate completely.

House dust mites do seem to be important in making asthma worse. Although their role in atopic eczema is less well established, they are worth taking seriously in some cases.

How do I know if my son is allergic to house dust mites?

It is easy to find evidence of allergy to house dust mites by subjecting your son to skin-prick testing, but the result may not be very useful. Many people with eczema have a positive reaction to house dust mites – and to many other allergens that do not seem to make their eczema worse. Many children without eczema also have positive reactions to house dust mites. If you suspect that house dust mites may be important in your son's eczema, it may be best to try some avoidance measures (see Chapter 4) rather than having the test done. The test itself involves putting on to the skin drops of liquid that either contains mite extract in saline (salt water) or is just saline on its own. The skin is then pricked with a needle through each drop, and the skin's reaction is tested. A strong reaction to mite extract compared with saline indicates a positive result.

I had a blood test at the hospital and have been told I am allergic to house dust mites. Is this a good test?

This is probably a RAST test, which detects antibodies in your blood that react to different things. The test is good at detecting an allergy, but the link between having the allergy and actually getting problems on your skin is sometimes less clear. It is certainly worth you trying all the avoidance measures (see Chapter 4). A RAST test is not able to detect general allergies as it is quite specific, so each test needs to focus on one possible cause or related groups of substances, for example dairy products, nuts or cats.

People keep telling me that the eczema on my hands is just a sign of stress. Is this true?

Stress is mentioned as a cause or trigger of many different diseases, not just ones that affect the skin. It is easy to generalise but difficult to be sure in any individual case. The best test may be to keep a diary of when your hands flare up and see whether this is related to times when you feel under stress. Some interesting work has been done looking at people's reaction to stress as a risk factor for developing eczema on the hands. It does seem that if you are someone who is more affected by stress and doesn't deal with it well, you do have a greater chance of developing hand eczema. This is interesting as it relates to some of the ideas in homeopathy, acupuncture and other complementary medical philosophies that take account of the type of person you are when choosing a treatment. To generalise a bit, the younger you are when you develop hand eczema and if patch tests are negative for allergy, the more likely you are to be affected by stress.

Is diet important?

During a recent bout of sickness and diarrhoea, my daughter's eczema almost disappeared. She ate hardly anything during this time. Could this mean that her eczema is related to the food she eats?

Unfortunately, this is not the likeliest explanation for the improvement in your daughter's eczema. Diet has not been shown to be a major factor in causing eczema, despite many people's view to the contrary. You have to remember that eczema fluctuates in severity all the time, often for reasons that we cannot explain. It is always tempting to look at 'what happened the day before' as the cause of a flare or an improvement, and doctors are no different from you in wanting a simple explanation.

Any infections (including tummy upsets) can improve eczema or cause a flare, presumably owing to the effect that they can have on the body's immune system or the fact that having a high temperature may make the skin more itchy. It is equally likely that your daughter's sickness had no effect on her eczema but that it was simply improving spontaneously at that time.

Could something in my son's diet be causing his eczema?

Although you don't say how old your son is, the answer is probably that his diet is not having an effect. Diet may be important in the initial triggering of eczema in infants with an inherited susceptibility, but it seems to have little to do with keeping eczema going or triggering it in older children. It is true that many parents, and indeed some doctors, think that diet is very important in eczema, but evidence from research studies over the past few years does not support this view. Life would be a lot easier if diet did have a major impact, but we have to believe the evidence from these well-conducted studies. We have used special diets in the past, but they are normally disappointing in terms of improving the eczema and are difficult to stick to, especially for children of school age.

Our advice to you is that if there is a clear history of your son's eczema always worsening after eating a certain food, it is worth a 3-month trial of excluding that food – after taking advice from a dietitian. If there is no improvement in his eczema after 3 months, that food should be gradually reintroduced. It cannot be overemphasised that all attempts at dietary manipulation should be made under the control of a dietitian to ensure that there is adequate calorie, protein, calcium and vitamin replacement. We have seen children with malnutrition and even rickets from unsupervised severe exclusion diets, and unfortunately they both still had bad eczema.

Will altering my diet during breast-feeding stop my baby from developing eczema? What else can I do to avoid triggering the condition?

Eczema is an inherited condition, but it is also influenced by environmental factors. We do not understand why it develops at a certain age in any one individual. There are important trigger factors, but little is known about them. It has been suggested that the early diet of a child, particularly an exposure to dairy products, might be important in triggering eczema.

There is scant evidence to support the idea that if you changed to a diet free from milk and eggs during breast-feeding, it might provide some protection against your baby developing eczema, especially if both you and the baby's father have a history of the condition. This view is still controversial, and we would not recommend such a diet routinely. It would certainly need to be done under the guidance of a dietitian.

Is breast-feeding better than bottle-feeding for helping to prevent my baby getting eczema?

This is a bit controversial now! The old answer was that the evidence seemed to suggest it was of benefit, although some research studies failed to show any advantage. Recently, however, a big study in New Zealand showed that breast-feeding was linked to a greater chance of a baby getting eczema than bottle-feeding. More research is needed before a definite answer can be given to this simple question as it relates to eczema. Breast-feeding does, however, have many other advantages, so we wouldn't yet go against the motto 'breast is best'.

I want to continue breast-feeding my baby, but the eczema on my nipples is making this very difficult. Have you any advice that could help?

Breast-feeding with eczema on the nipple or areolar tissue round it can be troublesome from time to time because this area can easily become infected with thrush, making it cracked and sore. Ask your doctor to examine your baby's mouth as well as your breasts as thrush may be present there too. There are topical creams that can be prescribed to resolve the infection.

During treatment, breast-feeding from the affected side should be temporarily stopped and expressing carried out instead, either manually or with the aid of an electric or hand pump. Your baby will be able to feed sufficiently from one breast only as the extra demand will increase the milk supply. Any expressed milk may be given to your baby or frozen for future use. As the skin heals, breast-feeding can be resumed, but care must be taken that your baby is well positioned and correctly attached on the breast at each feed to minimise any trauma or friction to the nipple. Further assistance with breast-feeding can be obtained from your local breast-feeding counsellor.

My baby has developed eczema. Could it be something to do with what I ate during pregnancy?

It sounds as though you are feeling guilty, as if your baby's eczema is your fault. There is no good evidence that what you eat during pregnancy has any effect on the subsequent development of eczema in a baby. Relax – it is not your 'fault'.

Are there any tests?

I have heard a lot about different allergy tests and am confused. My local supermarket offers tests of this kind, and a friend has also suggested an ELISA test. Can you give me any more information about these types of test and allergy tests in general?

'Allergy tests' mean different things to different people, and you will hear a lot of conflicting information about their use. Broadly speaking, there are two types of allergy test applicable to skin disease:

- patch tests;
- skin-prick tests (this type of testing can also be carried out on blood samples with an ELISA test, but both of these techniques are testing the same thing).

Patch tests look for evidence of contact eczema (also called dermatitis), such as is seen in allergy to nickel, chromate, rubber, dyes, glues or perfumes. This is a delayed allergy that sometimes develops after repeated exposure to a substance. Contact eczema is uncommon in children, perhaps because they have not had enough exposure to these allergens, so patch tests are not needed (or indeed helpful) in uncomplicated atopic eczema in childhood. Patch tests are complicated to do and interpret (they are carried out only by specialist dermatologists) but are useful in investigating certain types of eczema – such as isolated hand eczema, especially in people with certain jobs, for example hairdressers, builders and nurses.

Skin-prick tests (or ELISA tests) look for an immediate type of allergy (type 1 allergy). There are hundreds of allergens that can be used in these tests, but the common ones are pollens (grass and tree), dog fur, cat fur, house dust mite, egg, milk, fish and nuts. They can be useful in detecting relevant allergens in asthma, food intolerance and hay fever. They do not, however, provide much, if any, useful information in atopic eczema, and most experts in childhood eczema now realise this. The majority of children with eczema have multiple positive results to the skin-prick test, and these are difficult to interpret in any useful way. Children's skin seems hyperreactive to many substances. Although some doctors still do these tests, we believe that it is unjustified to inflict 15 pin-pricks or a blood test on a young child with atopic eczema if it is not going to provide any practical information in helping to manage the eczema. These tests do not help in deciding whether a certain food might make eczema worse and, if they are wrongly interpreted, can cause problems if nutritional foods are unnecessarily excluded.

I sent a piece of my hair away for testing and it came back with a whole list of foods that I am allergic to. My GP doesn't believe the result and says I should see an immunologist. Can't I just stop eating all those foods?

There is a great problem with the sort of testing you have had done. Often, there is very little science behind the test and the results, and we feel that the people doing the tests have a financial interest in the test being positive. Immunologists work much more with properly researched and what we call 'evidence-based' tests so can give more accurate results. If you tried to avoid the 'whole list of foods', your health would probably suffer greatly so it is not safe just to stop eating them. Any dietary modification should be carried out with advice, and perhaps supervision, from a dietitian.

Immunologists may need to play a bigger role in managing cases like yours in the future, especially when tests for 'intolerance' as opposed to true allergy are established and properly validated. To date, however, there are very few immunologists in the NHS, and waiting lists are long.

My doctor has refused to do allergy tests on my daughter – can I insist that these be done?

It sounds as though you and your doctor have a problem. Words like 'refuse' and 'insist' are very strong as you need to be able to discuss the investigation and treatment of your daughter's eczema in a calm way. If you read through the answers given above about allergy testing, it might help you to understand why such tests are not likely to change the way in which your daughter is treated. This is a very important concept, and doctors are often the worst offenders in carrying out tests unnecessarily. With eczema, it is very difficult to justify the pain inflicted on your daughter by having the tests done, and in today's tightly budgeted NHS we have to look at the cost of tests as well as treatment, and be able to justify the expense.

I have a leg ulcer but also seem to have developed eczema on my leg. Is this caused by the ulcer?

Having an ulcer does mean that the skin on your leg is weak and prone to damage so you are more likely to develop irritation and even allergies to the various treatments used for your ulcer. It is not therefore a direct effect but is a consequence of having the ulcer. The bandaging used to treat the ulcer occludes the skin and increases the likelihood of a reaction to creams or dressings under the bandages. You might need to have patch tests to check for allergies to substances being used to treat your ulcer.

Allergy problems

My eczema doesn't seem to behave as it should! I keep getting flares around my eyes and eyelids, and my GP can't explain why. I always use the same creams, which sometimes work and sometimes don't. Should I see a consultant?

This is a common presentation of any allergic contact eczema. Unusual patterns like this should always suggest the need for allergy testing. The skin around the eyes and on the eyelids is very sensitive, and one common cause of allergy is actually nail varnish. We are sure you are not applying nail varnish anywhere near your eyes, but you might be surprised how often you touch this area, and if you are wearing nail varnish this can cause a reaction. It could also be a reaction to any make-up you might use intermittently around the eyes, and you could also have developed an allergy to one of your treatments.

I recently had to go to hospital for patch-testing and found out I was allergic to nickel. I try to make sure I don't come into contact with it, but I still seem to get eczema. Is nickel eczema just from contact with it?

You have probably been given a list of metals that contain nickel, but it also occurs in many foods, which could be a reason for your eczema continuing. You could also have several different triggers for your eczema, not just nickel.

Cheap jewellery is not the only source of direct contact with nickel as it is unfortunately present in many common items made of, or containing, metal:

- clothes fastenings such as jeans studs, hooks and zips;
- other personal objects – cigarette lighters, wristwatches, key rings, keys, parts of spectacle frames and pens;
- household items such as drawer and cupboard handles, kitchen utensils, toasters, etc.

- silver coins.

The list could almost be endless so only a few examples are given here. The nickel content of some foods comes from natural sources or from the way in which they are prepared. This is usually only a problem if you have a severe reaction to nickel, which often shows up as a blistering eczema (pompholyx) on the hands. Avoid canned foods, and use aluminium or stainless steel utensils when cooking. A dietitian could give you a list of foods to avoid, which will include asparagus, oysters, herrings (other fish are OK), mushrooms, onions, tomatoes and rhubarb.

Food and oral medication

Is it worth having tests for food intolerance? I have recently read about this testing and about claims that most people get better after testing, although nothing has been published. Is it worth doing?

These tests are being developed but, at the time of writing, have not been fully evaluated or validated. This process is very important if the tests are to be used to change treatments or dietary habits. Tests need to be accurate and repeatable – this means that they should give the same result no matter how many times you are tested before having any treatment so that changes in the results can be believed.

Could I sometimes be allergic to dairy products and sometimes not? I notice that my skin sometimes seems to get worse when I drink milk?

One possible explanation may be that the lining of the gut can become inflamed when eczema is severe, and larger proteins than normal can get through. These larger proteins may trigger an immune response and cause further exacerbations, but once the eczema has settled, the gut returns to normal and the larger proteins are kept out.

My asthma flared up recently, and my doctor told me to stop taking aspirin or Nurofen. Could these also have been causing my eczema?

Some people with atopic diseases such as eczema, asthma and hay fever are sensitive to the effects of 'salicylates'. These are naturally occurring substances very similar to aspirin, which was derived originally from willow bark. Nurofen and other 'non-steroidal anti-inflammatory drugs' have a similar action to aspirin and can share some of its potential reactions. This appears to be much more of a problem with asthma than eczema. Salicylates tend to give an urticaria (hives) rather than eczema, but they could be a factor for you.

Miscellaneous

I work in a sawmill and get eczema on my hands. This is put down to wear and tear, but recently I got eczema on my face, which I think is also worse at work. Could it be something in the air?

You could have a combination of a physical contact irritant eczema from the wear and tear, and an allergic form from natural resins in the wood or agents used to treat the wood. If the ventilation is poor and the atmosphere you work in is heavy with dust, you could well get an allergic reaction on your face. Talk to your GP about a referral for patch-testing.

My parents have always recommended massaging mustard oil into the arms and legs of our children to help with strong bone growth. I have a 3-year-old daughter with eczema and am worried that this might make it worse. What should I do?

We have come across the practice of using mustard oil on the skin in families from Africa and the Indian subcontinent. There isn't any scientific evidence that this practice helps with bone growth, but many people are strong believers in it. It is important to try to respect cultural practices as they may be helpful, or at least not harmful, to eczema. For example, many West Indian and Indian parents use olive oil or aloe vera cream as a moisturiser, and these seem to be beneficial. Some Nigerian families use hibiscus flower water on the skin; although we are not sure that this helps, it certainly does not seem to make things worse.

Mustard oil, however, is *very* irritant to the broken skin of eczema and will nearly always make it worse. Because of this, we strongly advise you not to use it. A balanced diet with plenty of calcium and exercise will ensure good bone growth. You will have to explain to your parents politely, but firmly, that mustard oil would make their grand-daughter's eczema worse and that she is growing into a healthy girl without it.

All my children have suffered with bad cradle cap and nappy rash. Why is this, and why did they all get better after a few months?

It sounds as though all your children had seborrhoeic eczema. In a mild form, this is almost universal in babies. It is probably caused by a transfer of hormones (androgens) from mother to baby just before birth. These hormones act to stimulate the grease glands (sebaceous glands) of the skin, making them overactive. They are usually inactive in children until puberty. This hormonal stimulation causes the greasy scaling so typical of this type of eczema. The scalp and nappy area are commonly affected – hence the usual presentation with cradle cap and nappy rash.

As babies do not make these hormones themselves, and because the transferred hormones are soon broken down and inactivated, the problem of seborrhoeic eczema resolves completely on its own in a few months.

I suffer with eczema on my hands, which I think is made worse by work, although I work in an office and don't handle any chemicals. Could there be another explanation?

Your work environment might be a problem as the low-humidity from air-conditioning can dry out anybody's skin, and this will be a bigger problem for you. It will show up as redness and scaling. Repeated friction from handling papers or other materials can also be a problem, leading to a physical eczema that will differ in looking less red, but dry and thickened.

I have just come back from holiday with the most awful eczema. My doctor says it is photo-dermatitis and might be due to a new sunscreen. Will I ever be able to go on holiday again?

Yes, you will. A type of allergic contact eczema whose cause involves natural or artificial ultraviolet light is quite rare but may be on the increase. Sunscreens are the most commonly reported culprits (photo-allergens), but they are always used in the sun! Other common photo-allergens are fragrances, topical non-steroidal anti-inflammatory drugs and some antibacterial creams. You might need to be referred to hospital for a special form of patch-testing that uses ultraviolet light to mimic the conditions in which you reacted – this is called photo-patch-testing. This should allow the dermatologist to tell you what sunscreens you can safely use.

I first started having eczema around my fingernails, which might have been due to the false nails I wore. I then got it in my hair – have I transferred it to my scalp from my fingers when I wash my hair?

Eczema is not a contagious disease so you will not have transferred it to your scalp. As you have developed eczema around your fingernails from an allergy to the acrylics in false nails, you do have a risk of developing eczema elsewhere. Once you have an allergy to something, any part of your skin can react in the same way, so if you washed your hair with the false nails on, this might have been enough contact to start the eczema. There may, however, have been a different trigger for your scalp eczema, such as a different shampoo or hair treatment.

One of the residents in the nursing home where I work had scabies. I caught it and had treatment, but my doctor says I now have eczema. Does scabies cause eczema?

It is very common to have a rash that looks just like eczema after scabies (an infestation with little mites that burrow into the skin) as you will have developed an allergy to the dead mites and their waste matter. Standard eczema treatments should settle it down over a few weeks, but it will leave your skin in a vulnerable state for the next few months so soaps and other products that might not have bothered you before could cause a problem. Take good care of your skin and it should all settle down and not trouble you again.

I think something in my garden makes my eczema worse. Any clues you could give me would be welcome as I don't want to give up gardening.

There are many things in the garden that can cause skin problems, some of which are quite dramatic, with acute blistering rashes from a combination of plant juices and the sun. It sounds as though you already have eczema that gets worse when you garden, and this could be due to several factors. The very act of using your hands outdoors, with rubbing, hard work and the extra washing required, can cause problems in terms of physical irritants. Some plants are associated with eczema; these include chrysanthemums, which tend to give a thickened, dry eczema on exposed parts, and tulip bulbs, which classically give rise to a fingertip eczema. The pollen in the air near chrysanthemums can cause the reaction so you don't even have to be in direct contact.

3
Complications and what can make eczema worse

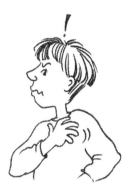

Introduction

Eczema is a condition that has a tendency to flare up and settle. It will often seem manageable and tolerable, but there may well be times when the skin becomes more red and inflamed, with weeping areas and general background dryness. The chapters on treatment will help to give guidance on managing such flares, so this chapter will concentrate on some factors that may tend to make eczema worse or that may trigger a flare. Eczema can vary in severity from one individual to the next: some readers will find that they have eczema affecting their whole body, whereas others may have it only on specific areas such as the hands, legs or scalp. A 'flare' describes a worsening of the eczema. An acute eczema flare can cause you to feel generally unwell, which may in some cases require hospitalisation, but the majority of cases can be self-managed at home.

There are some triggers that can make existing eczema worse even though they do not cause it to start in normal skin. The reason for this is that our skin acts as a barrier, but when it is inflamed and dry, it stops working so well. Imagine your skin as a brick wall with faulty cement between the bricks: gaps then appear, and items can pass through the wall. This allows water to leak out of the body and the skin to be rather oversensitive and susceptible to things it comes into contact with. This might be items such as woolly clothes, perfumes or cosmetics, or microscopic factors that act as triggers, for example bacterial or viral infections.

Complications

Bacterial infection

My son's eczema became much worse and wasn't improving with the creams. The GP said it was infected and gave him a course of antibiotics. What caused this infection, and can it be dangerous?

We all have micro-organisms on our skin called *Staphylococcus aureus*. In eczematous skin, the barrier function is not working effectively, and micro-organisms that come into contact with the skin are more likely to initiate an inflammatory response. It is thought that there are more *Staphylococcus* organisms on eczematous skin, and this can lead to clinical infection.

A bacterial infection on the skin generally has a localised effect, seen as redness, weeping, crusting and odour. If extensive areas are affected, this can lead to symptoms of general malaise and fever arising from a toxic reaction to the chemicals released as part of the process of fighting the infection in the skin. There is evidence that a toxin produced by *Staphylococcus aureus* can cause a flare of eczema elsewhere on the skin so it is often treated with antibiotics by mouth to try to prevent this. If you or your son recognises that there is an infection present and seeks treatment from your GP, you should find that it settles quickly with no danger to your son.

My daughter's eczema is raw and weepy. Does this mean that it is infected?

Not necessarily. An acute eczema does present as inflamed weeping skin, which can be made worse by scratching and can then become infected. The more chronic, or long term, an area of eczema becomes, the more likely it is to be dry and thickened. If your daughter had chronic eczema that suddenly became wet and weepy, it would be quite likely that an infection had triggered this change. Signs of clinical infection are pain, swelling, odour and pus. As previously mentioned, eczematous skin may harbour the bacterium *Staphylococcus aureus*; if the skin appears to be infected, a swab can be taken to identify the bacteria responsible and the antibiotics that will work.

When I saw the specialist recently, she took swabs from my nose and skin. Later, she wrote to say I had an infection and gave me some nose cream. Why treat the nose for a skin infection?

Bacteria that can cause infection on the skin can sometimes be harboured in the nose. If we see people who have been troubled with recurrent flares and infections of the skin, we will often carry out a nose swab to see whether they are a carrier of *Staphylococcus aureus*. As in your case, a positive swab can be treated effectively with a nasal ointment called mupirocin (Bactroban). This will reduce the bacterial count and prevent further infective flares. It seems that bacteria living inside the nose often survive despite courses of antibiotics given by mouth so this extra treatment is necessary to help to prevent a recurrence. In difficult cases, we often ask for similar swabs to be taken from other people living with you in case they are harbouring the bacteria. Like you, they will not have any signs of infection in the nose – we call this 'carriage' as the bacteria are just being carried inside the nose without causing local infection.

I have quite widespread eczema that has been good recently, but I have developed what looks like a shaving rash on my legs! Can I still apply my creams?

It sounds as though you are doing your best to treat your eczema and keep your skin in good condition with moisturisers. In eczema management, we use very greasy moisturisers as these help to manage the dryness of the skin, but they can cause the small hair follicles on the skin's surface to become blocked. Once the follicles are blocked, folliculitis (an inflammation of the hair follicle) can develop, which tends to look like a shaving rash. This can commonly be seen after using paste bandages or when the weather has been hot and sticky. You can still use creams to treat the eczema, but it would be helpful to follow the guidance below to avoid further bouts of folliculitis:

- Use a lighter, cream-based moisturiser (see Table 2 in Chapter 4).

- Smooth the moisturiser on to the skin in a wiping action, following the same direction that the hairs grow (i.e. like stroking a cat). There is no need to massage or rub cream into the skin as this just pushes the cream up into the hair follicle.

- If a topical steroid is being used, it should be in a cream rather than an ointment base.

- It might be useful to leave bandaging off until the problem has settled.

If the areas of folliculitis become more widespread, inflamed and painful, they may have become infected. Seek advice from your doctor if this happens as oral antibiotics are sometimes needed.

Eczema herpeticum, warts and molluscum

I was diagnosed with eczema herpeticum, which cleared up quickly after treatment with aciclovir. Is there more information on this condition?

Eczema herpeticum is a term used for a severe, widespread skin infection with the herpes virus that occasionally occurs in people with eczema. Herpes infections are usually localised, causing a few blisters or a cold sore on the lip. Eczema herpeticum shows much more widespread blistering of the skin and also 'punched-out' sores, which look like little holes in the skin. Typically, the condition involves the face, but it can occur anywhere on the body. Multiple punched-out, crusted lesions around a patch of eczema should make you suspicious. It is sometimes, but not always, associated with a high temperature, and if this was the case with you, you probably felt very unwell. In rare cases, it can be a very severe infection, especially if it is not recognised and treated – and it may require hospital admission. Although it is said to have caused death on one or two occasions, we believe that this is rare because most individuals or their carers will seek medical help before such a risk arises. As you have found out, treatment involves a simple course of tablets taken by mouth.

Eczema herpeticum is thought to occur because some people with eczema do not fight off viruses affecting the skin very quickly, and the scratching and skin damage helps to spread the virus. It is possible to suffer from it more that once, but it seems that the first bout of infection is often the worst, with much less chance of it becoming serious during recurrences.

Are warts more common with children with eczema?

Viral warts are very common in all children, especially on the hands and feet. They are often noticed more readily in children with eczema because such children are already being seen by doctors about their eczema and are having their skin examined more frequently. Warts are not necessarily more common in children – or adults – with eczema, but there is some evidence that they become more numerous once they have been caught. A wart is actually an virus infection in the skin so scratching will help to spread it around the skin. In addition, it is thought that skin affected by eczema is not as efficient as 'normal' skin at getting rid of viral infections so this may also cause them to spread more easily. Warts are 'self-limiting', which means that they will eventually disappear with no treatment even in the presence of eczema. This can be as soon as a couple of months or stretch up to a few years for some people, and having eczema does not mean that they will last any longer.

My daughter has had eczema for 3 years. She recently developed a new rash, which our doctor said was molluscum. What is this?

Molluscum, also called molluscum contagiosum, is a type of tiny wart in the skin that looks rather like small, translucent blisters. These are caused by an infection with a poxvirus. Some people refer to them as water warts, although they are in fact solid. They are dome shaped and often have a small depression or punctum on the top. Molluscum is common in children and young adults, and is more frequently seen in patients with eczema, perhaps because the process of scratching causes the virus to spread. As with warts, the blisters eventually clear on their own, which is just as well because treatment can be painful – for example, using liquid nitrogen spray to freeze them off. They are not serious and can be safely left alone.

I have lightish olive skin and notice that I get darker areas persisting even when my eczema has cleared. Why is this?

It sounds as though you have had a change in the pigment in your skin. Episodes of inflammation in the skin from eczema and other causes can lead to pigment changes, leaving the skin lighter or darker. We call this process post-inflammatory hypo- (if lighter) or hyper- (if darker) pigmentation. The darker your skin is to start with, the more likely it is to get darker still. Except in a few cases, the effect is not permanent, although it can last for several months or longer depending on how bad your eczema is. Please don't try treating these areas with any lightening creams you might see advertised as these can be irritant to the skin, make your eczema flare up and make the problem worse!

It can be serious

My daughter had to be admitted urgently to hospital because her eczema was bad and she became very floppy and ill. I thought eczema was 'just a skin disease'.

It sounds as though your daughter's eczema has been very severe. As you say, many people see eczema simply as 'just a skin disease', but the skin is the body's largest organ, and it is responsible for maintaining temperature control and fluid balance. If a considerable area of skin becomes inflamed and weepy, as seen in eczema flares, this role becomes more and more difficult to maintain, leading to water and heat loss from the body. The water loss can occur through wet, weepy areas of skin or simply via the process of evaporation from the hot, inflamed skin.

When the skin becomes hot and red all over, this is known as erythroderma, and urgent treatment is necessary. This is particularly important in children, who can very quickly become ill from dehydration as they have a larger area of skin in relation to their body size so the potential for losing too much water is greater. Although the skin is not damaged or scarred in the long term from severe problems like this, the effects of losing heat and water can be as bad as if your daughter had suffered widespread burns. This problem is not confined to children: although it is rare, anyone with a tendency to widespread eczema (usually atopic in type) could suffer this type of complication.

What can make eczema worse?

My symptoms of eczema seems to be much worse now as soon as I get home from work. As soon as I get in, I start scratching for no reason, and it gets worse over the evening and in my sleep. Why is this happening?

The pattern of scratching and irritation you describe could arise for a number of reasons. First, consider your home environment: for example, do you keep your home very warm? The use of central heating can create a dry atmosphere; this plus the heat can act as a trigger to irritation in eczema so it is best to keep your home cool if possible. This might not be tolerated quite as well by others you share the house with, but it will be helpful in reducing your irritation. Also consider whether other factors at home – for example, animal dander or cigarette smoke – could be causing the exacerbation. Your home differs from the environment at work as it comprises more carpeting, curtains and soft furnishings, all of which are a potential haven for house dust mites. Measures to reduce house dust mites (as described in Chapter 4) might help your eczema so might be worth trying for a couple of months to see whether they have an effect.

Just being relaxed at home could be part of the problem too as you are probably busy and distracted at work – so although you might get the itchy sensation, you might not have the opportunity to scratch. Once at home, you might feel more 'free' to scratch, and there are fewer distractions to blur the itch sensation. This can progress to the point at which you might have developed a habit of scratching as soon as you get home. Once an itch–scratch cycle is established, it can become habitual. If you feel that this could be a possibility, you may find the advice at the end of Chapter 4 helpful.

Since I have developed eczema, I have been told not to use soap, but I don't really feel clean unless I have used soap. Can you suggest one that I can use?

Soaps have an alkaline base and as such have a drying, irritant effect on the skin. When we use a soap to cleanse the skin, it removes not only the dirt, but also the protective grease produced by the skin to maintain the barrier function. We only have to look at the hands of people who do a lot of washing-up and cleaning to see how irritant soap can be so it should be avoided by anyone with eczema. By soap, we mean anything that creates lather or bubbles so bubble bath and shower gel should also be avoided. A soap substitute, such as aqueous cream or emulsifying ointment, should be used instead; this will still have an effective cleansing effect on your skin. There are also some more expensive soap-free lotions that you might find easier to use – they even come in containers like shower gel. If you are set on using soap, try to limit it to specific areas such as your armpits and choose a pH-neutral variety that is non-perfumed and has added moisturising creams.

Can you give me some advice about diet and eczema?

A number of research studies have examined the role of diet in atopic eczema so this answer really only applies if you have this type. These studies have looked at exclusion of diary products, chicken, wheat, flavourings and additives. Some studies seem to indicate a link, but many of the newer studies do not show any relationship. You have to remember that all studies of eczema are difficult, for three reasons:

- First, eczema fluctuates in severity, regardless of any treatment given.

- Second, eczema spontaneously resolves in most children as they get older.

- Finally, it is difficult to accurately quantify or score the severity of eczema.

Studies have to take all these factors into account and ideally use a placebo group who receive no active treatment. The placebo group is important because one must know how many people would improve even though they are not getting any of the specific treatments being assessed in the trial.

This all seems rather confusing, but the most recent studies have been well conducted and have used placebo groups. They have looked mainly at dairy-free diets and very severe exclusion diets, such as elemental diets in which only a few types of food are allowed. The results have shown that dietary changes do not usually cause an improvement in eczema after the age of 1 year. There was a possible benefit from a dairy-free diet in children under 1 year old, but the effect was so small that, statistically, this might have occurred by chance. All studies have revealed that it is difficult for families to stick to special diets, especially when children go to school, parties, etc. We do not routinely advise dietary manipulation as a way of treating eczema. If you are convinced that one food or a group of related foods is important in making your eczema worse, you should only try and change your diet with the help of a dietitian.

Would you ever use a diet?

Yes, we would occasionally consider a dairy-free diet in a child less than 1 year old if other conventional treatments were not working well. In addition, if there were a clear-cut history of a certain food making the eczema worse every time it was consumed, we would consider a 3-month exclusion trial.

To ensure that adequate nutrition is provided, a dietitian should supervise any dietary approach. A dietitian can also give invaluable advice on which foods to use and where to obtain them. Do not try to follow diets listed in magazines or shown on the television as there is the potential to develop a regime that does not completely exclude all the relevant food, and there is also a risk of undernourishing the child.

At the end of the 3-month exclusion, the food thought to be at fault should be reintroduced. If the eczema does not come back, it may be that it was only a temporary problem or that the food was not making the eczema worse. If the eczema returns, the exclusion diet should be restarted as the final 'proof' needs to come from demonstrating that the exclusion works a second time. Even in this case, the problem rarely persists for more than a year or so.

We wish that diet were more important in eczema as it would provide an easy and safe approach to therapy. Our general experience has, however, shown that diets are extremely hard work and are often disappointing in terms of any impact they have on eczema.

I have eczema and am very allergic to peanuts. Are these two conditions related?

No, they are probably not directly related. Nuts, especially peanuts, are well known for causing a severe allergic reaction, called anaphylaxis, characterised by swelling of the lips and face, vomiting, difficulty breathing, a widespread nettle rash and even collapse. The incidence of this appears to be increasing, and the allergy is lifelong, unlike many other childhood food intolerances.

There is a growing feeling that children, especially those with an 'atopic tendency', should avoid eating peanuts, and to a lesser extent other nuts, until late childhood. This may prevent nut allergy developing but has nothing to do with the causes of eczema. You should make sure that you carry a card or wear a bracelet to let anyone know that you have this problem in case you are so badly affected that you cannot speak.

Should I remove foods containing colourings and additives from my daughter's diet?

Unless there is a very strong link with her eczema, i.e. every time these foods are consumed the eczema becomes worse, we do not think that this is necessary. Colourings and additives may be important with some children with another disorder called urticaria or hives, but the link with eczema is very tenuous. In practice, they are extremely difficult to avoid as they seem to be added to so many foods favoured by children. It may be helpful to discuss this further with a dietitian before embarking on such an exclusion diet.

Is there anything else we can do to stop the eczema getting worse?

Apart from following the advice in the chapter on treatment, there are some general measures that can be of benefit. As with other bits of general advice in this book, the measures may apply much more to people with an atopic type of eczema:

- Avoid any pets with furry or hairy coats, such as rabbits, hamsters, cats, dogs and horses. We don't advise getting rid of existing pets, but you might want to consider not replacing them when they die.

- Clothes and bedding should be of cotton or even silk as these are less irritant than wool and synthetic materials.

- Keep fingernails cut short, and consider wearing cotton gloves or mittens at night.

- Try to use a non-biological washing powder and rinse clothes thoroughly after washing to remove traces of soap powder. It might be useful to use an extra rinse cycle on the washing machine.

- Pollen can sometimes make eczema worse. Adult eczema sufferers can ask a relative or friend to cut the grass; if your child is affected, cut the grass in the evening after he or she has gone to bed.

- Wear cotton gloves when doing housework such as vacuuming, polishing or dusting, keep the room well ventilated, and if your child has eczema, ask him or her to stay out of the room you are cleaning.

- Keep cool; sweat can irritate the skin, leading to intensely itchy, dry, eczematous skin.

- Avoid handling or preparing irritant foods such as citrus fruits, onions, chillies, raw vegetables (especially tomatoes) and salty food.

- Cigarette smoke can be an irritant to eczema so encourage smokers to keep their habit outside the home.

I have been recently advised that my daughter's eczema is aggravated by teething, smoke and cat or dog hair. She is 18 months old. Could you please advise on such claims – she hasn't had any tests?

It depends a bit on who is giving you this advice and whether it is general or specific. Teething has been reported as causing flares of eczema on the face in young children, but this could be related to the increased dribbling causing irritation around the mouth rather than to any direct effect of teething. Smoke is irritant to the skin so this is good advice – try to make sure that your daughter is not exposed to any smoke.

Cat and dog hair can be a problem, and this is usually a direct allergic effect so could show up on a blood test. It is very unfair to make young children have blood tests as you may already have a feeling that the family pet is causing a problem. It is interesting that it is not cat hair itself that causes the problem but something in the cat's saliva, which coats the hairs after all the washing that cats do. With dogs, the allergen is in the hair itself. Try to keep the pet out of your daughter's bedroom, and keep a play mat handy to put down on carpets that may have pet hair on them.

4
First-line treatment

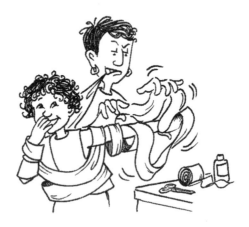

Introduction

The treatment of eczema should reflect the needs of the individual and their eczema. The extent of the eczema and the areas affected will influence the choice of treatment. Although there are a variety of different treatment approaches, first-line therapy usually involves a topical skin-care regime in which creams or ointments are applied directly to the skin. This usually involves the regular use of moisturisers with the addition of topical steroids as an active treatment when needed.

Skin-care regimes such as these are the mainstay of eczema management, but they can be messy, fiddly and time-consuming, leading to a potential underuse or misuse of treatment and difficulties of 'sticking' to the regime. With a chronic condition such as eczema, the results of treatment are not always instant or clearly visible, hence it can be difficult to maintain motivation and concordance with therapy. It is the skill of the doctor or nurse to enthuse, inform and educate those with eczema so that they can make informed treatment decisions in partnership with health-care professionals. This is why we use the term 'concordance' instead of the more old-fashioned term 'compliance' as it reflects some agreement on the type of treatment regime chosen. In addition, it is important to be aware of other sources of information, such as the National Eczema Society.

Overall, the key thing to consider with the management of eczema is to be realistic about treatment expectations. Eczema is a chronic condition, and therefore the aim of treatment is improved management and maintenance. Clearance may be attained in the short term, but a cure is not possible. When deciding on the mode of treatment, one must consider the fine balance between clearance and the potential of side-effects of the treatment. To better illustrate this point, think of a couple of different scenarios: for a child a realistic expectation might be to control the eczema at a level that does not interfere with social, psychological or physical development, whereas with adults the goal may be to maintain eczema at a level that does not interfere with a desirable quality of life. This can be much more realistic and achievable than always aiming for completely clear skin.

No matter how well eczema is controlled, there will always be the occasion when a flare is experienced. The nature of eczema is to fluctuate: a flare is not an indication that treatment has failed but just an indication to step up a gear to tackle a more severe presentation. It is therefore helpful to think of first-line eczema treatment as having two phases. The first is a maintenance phase consisting of a weaker treatment regime that will continue as long as the eczema has the potential to cause problems; the second is a stronger set of creams to use in the short term when the condition flares. A recent study of attitudes to eczema treatment interviewed 200 patients across Europe, with the following findings:

- 75% of patients/carers said that being able to control the eczema effectively would be the single most important improvement to their quality of life;

- 55% admitted to worrying about the next flare (36% sometimes worried, 19% *always* worried);

- patients with moderate eczema spent an average of 97 days each year in a flare, whereas for those with severe eczema the figure was 146 days;

- 66% of patients/carers used topical steroids only as a last resort; 58% restricted their use of topical steroids to certain body areas owing to concern about side-effects, and 39% used them less frequently than their doctor recommended, for the same reason;

- 67% of patients/carers said that their preferred treatment option was to apply a non-steroid treatment as early as possible to prevent a flare.

Topical treatments

Moisturisers and emollients

I have just been told I have eczema – what sort of creams will I have to use?

You will need to get used to using regular topical treatments – this means creams and ointments that you apply on to your skin rather than tablets you might take by mouth. A triple therapy approach is used, which entails:

- avoiding soaps by using a regime of soap substitutes and bath emollients to wash;

- regular use of a moisturiser;

- intermittent use of the weakest possible topical steroid.

My mother-in-law says I shouldn't bath my daughter more than once a week because this will make her eczema worse. Is this true?

No, bathing and cleansing the skin is a very important part of the skin care regime, so we would disagree with your mother-in-law. Having an emollient bath daily allows skin scale and crust to gently lift away without damaging the skin beneath. In addition, it enables old creams and ointments to be removed from the skin, and the process of cleansing will also reduce the bacterial count on the skin surface and thus reduce the chance of infection. Furthermore, the bath can be a comforting and fun experience for your daughter.

To get the best out of bathing, follow the key tips below:

- Always have the bath water cool or warm, never hot, as this will cause the skin to feel hot, dry and irritated after the bath.

- Avoid bubble bath and soap; these have an irritant and drying effect on the skin.

- Use a medicated bath oil. This will contain emulsifying agents, which allow the oil to contact the skin and prevent further drying.

- Use a soap substitute such as aqueous cream or emulsifying ointment, which will cleanse the skin effectively without drying. Note that when you scoop the emulsifying ointment from the pot, it will look like lard; with encouragement, it can make a rich, creamy mixture to wash with. Take it in your wet hands and work your hands together, add a little more water, and then in a few seconds it will change from an ointment to a cream.

- Have fun! Try to make emulsifying bubbles or aqueous cream sharks. Try to make bubble bath by running the tap over a pot of greasy emollient, and let siblings/partners in the bath too if the eczema is not wet or infected. For children, life without bubble bath can be difficult so try putting some bath emollient in a washed-out favourite bubble bath bottle and see if it is better accepted.

- Take care not to slip!
- Limit bathing to 10–15 minutes as beyond this your skin will start to dry.
- On getting out of the bath, pat the skin dry, but avoid vigorous rubbing, which could develop into scratching.
- After bathing is an ideal time to use a moisturiser; apply it liberally.

What are pH-neutral soaps, and are they better?

Normal soaps have an alkaline base so they have a high pH and tend to have a dry and irritant effect on the skin. A soap that is pH-neutral has a lower pH and is therefore less irritant. If you feel it necessary to use soap, this type is preferable, but overall it is best to use a soap substitute if you have eczema as this will cleanse the skin effectively without drying it.

Are there any differences between the bath oils used in eczema?

It is important to realise that by 'bath oil' we refer to medicinal oils rather than baby oil or olive oil. Medicinal oils contain emulsifying agents so that when they are added to the water, it turns an opaque colour as the oils mix with the water rather than floating on top of it; they thus have a therapeutic effect.

Many of the medicinal oils are very similar, but there are some differences in the base oil. Most are based on liquid paraffin, but some contain soya oil (Balneum) or wheat oil (Aveeno). The other factor is the percentage of oil: oils can occasionally feel very occlusive on the skin, and if that feeling is unpleasant it can be helpful to choose bath oil with a lower percentage of oil. This is a highly individual choice, and it might be worth trying a few alternatives before deciding on a regular bath emollient that you or your child feels happy with.

In addition, some bath oils contain additives, as shown in Table 1, such as antiseptics or antipruritic (anti-itch) agents. Antiseptics are useful as they reduce the bacterial count on the skin if recurrent skin infection has been a problem.

Table 1 Bath oils commonly used in eczema

Manufacturer	Name
Bristol-Myers Squibb	Alpha Keri Bath Oil
J&J	Aveeno (with oatmeal)
Crookes	Balneum, Balneum Plus
Sankyo	Cetraben
Dermal	Dermalo, Dermol 600, Emulsiderm
Schering-Plough	Diprobath
Crookes	E45
Ferndale	Hydromol Emollient
Stiefel	Oilatum, Oilatum Plus, Oilatum Fragrance Free

My 3-year-old daughter likes to drink her bath water! Is this dangerous?

Most toddlers seem to drink the bath water on occasions, and in small quantities this does not seem to be harmful, even if you are using a bath oil. Having special toys to play with in the bath, such as a duck or other plastic toys, can distract them from drinking the water. Bath time should be fun for children, but obviously there are a few hazards to avoid. Always use a non-slip bath mat to prevent accidents, and, as with any other medications, keep all skin-care products out of reach of children – preferably in a high, locked cupboard.

What is the difference between a moisturiser and an emollient?

There is no difference. 'Emollient' sounds somewhat more medical, but these words are interchangeable.

My main problem is that my skin dries out, leaving me itchy all over and red in a lot of places. I have tried non-steroid creams such as such as E45 and Diprobase cream, but neither helps.

By non-steroid creams, we presume you mean emollients or moisturisers: these play a key part in the management of eczema. Our skin normally acts as an effective barrier, reducing water loss from the skin and protecting us against things in our surroundings that we come into contact with. In eczema, this barrier is not working effectively so by applying emollients to the skin you will re-create the barrier function. You describe your skin as dry and itchy despite the use of creams. This poor control of symptoms could be related to the frequency and amount of cream you have used, or the moisturiser you have used may just not be greasy enough.

First, let's think of your moisturising regime. Ideally, the emollient should be applied at least two or three times daily, more often if the skin feels dry between applications. Remember that the role of an emollient is to prevent dryness, so do not allow the skin to become dry and scaly before you apply more. When applying your emollient, try to remember the following:

- Smooth the emollient in a downward direction, in the same direction as the hair growth.

- Do not rub it in vigorously as this stimulates itching; instead, smooth it on to the skin and it will soon soak in.

- Aim to see the skin glisten, and reapply the emollient frequently.

- Develop a regime of washing, moisturising and dressing that works well for you.

The regular use of a moisturiser will flatten out skin surface irregularities and improve flexibility so cracks and splits are less likely and the skin feels more comfortable.

Second, it might be worth reviewing the moisturiser you are using: if you are having to reapply it very frequently and your skin still feels dry, you may need a greasier base. Everyone is an individual and unfortunately there is no one moisturiser to suit all, so it is sometimes worth experimenting with different moisturisers until you find one that suits you. If you pay for prescriptions, this can get very expensive unless you have a prepayment certificate (see Chapter 11), so ask your GP or nurse if they have any sample bottles you could try first.

I have had both ointment and cream emollients prescribed for my eczema. Is one better than the other?

Generally speaking, a greasy emollient is better. Emollients are used to re-create the barrier function of the skin, and a greasy ointment will provide this most effectively as it creates an occlusive layer on the skin surface. You may ask why, if grease is best, there are so many other moisturisers available. This is because some people find the greasy ointments difficult to tolerate as they dislike being hot and sticky, and ointments can leave grease marks on clothing and soft furnishings in the home. An alternative is to use creams, which are water based and easily absorbed. As there is less oil in creams, these need to be applied more frequently to maintain the skin in a well-moisturised state. An advantage is that they provide a cooling effect once applied to the skin as the water evaporates away (which is useful for hot itchy skin).

Table 2 demonstrates the range of emollients available; the choice depends on your eczema as well as personal choice. If the eczema is very dry, try to use an ointment or a greasy cream. If you have weepy eczema, a cream is better as the ointment will float on the surface and be easily rubbed off. Overall, the best emollient is the one you feel comfortable using and is effective. Furthermore, you do not have to restrict yourself to one emollient: you may, for example, want a light lotion or cream for your face and thick grease for your feet. A useful regime is to use a cream in the day and an ointment at night. Again, it is worth seeing whether you can get hold of any small sample tubes to try at home.

Table 2 Some commonly used emollients, although others are available

Criteria for choice	Emollients – listed from light creams to greasy ointments
Easily applied, well tolerated. Contain preservatives, so observe for sensitivity to these. Creams have a high water content so can be cooling on hot, erythematous skin	Aqueous cream BP* E45 cream* Ultrabase Aveeno cream Cetraben
Greasier creams providing an effective barrier for moisture loss. Easily applied and well tolerated	Diprobase cream* Oilatum cream* Unguentum M* Neutrogena dermatological cream
A thicker base, but still water soluble, so can be used as soap substitutes. Not as easy to apply but offer an effective barrier without a wet/oily feel	Epaderm* Hydromol ointment* Emulsifying ointment BP*
Ointment base, easy to apply. May need a covering as they leave the skin greasy. Ideal for very dry and hyperkeratotic areas. Can be occlusive, causing a hot uncomfortable feeling, and may cause folliculitis	Dermamist Doublebase gel Diprobase ointment White soft paraffin/liquid paraffin 50/50
Emollients with specific properties	
Dermol 500 lotion* and Dermol cream	Antibacterial – useful with infected/excoriated eczema and methicillin-resistant *Staphylococcus aureus* (MRSA)
Aquadrate, Calmurid and Eucerin	Contain urea, a hydrating agent. Are useful for scaly conditions but may cause stinging
Balneum Plus	Contains urea and lauromacrogols, which have a local antipruritic action

*Emollients suitable for use as soap substitutes. They can also be used as moisturisers unless a lighter or greasier moisturiser is preferred. As a general rule, the drier the skin, the greasier the moisturiser needs to be.

I have always used aqueous cream as a moisturiser on my face, but last time I visited my GP he suggested stopping using it and finding an alternative. Why is this?

Aqueous cream has been commonly used as a moisturiser, but recent studies have found that some of the additives used in some formulations of aqueous cream can cause contact sensitivity and/or irritant reactions on the skin. It is for this reason that we would advise against aqueous cream being used as a leave-on moisturiser, although it can still be used as a soap substitute.

Steroids

My doctor has given me various creams, none of which works. Some of the steroid creams calm the area but only for short periods. Should I go back and ask for a new cream?

Before you go back for more cream, let's review what you have already been given and how you have used it. Using a skin-care regime and building it into your daily lifestyle is very important. As you mention, steroid creams can calm inflammation, but they are only one aspect of the regime and, to be effective, they need to be used in conjunction with an effective emollient. It is important to apply the emollient first and allow it to absorb for about 20 minutes before applying the topical steroid. This means that the steroid will be applied to a moisturised base and will be absorbed more readily.

It is also important to consider how much cream you are applying. Emollients are designed to be used liberally and frequently on all areas and as such should be prescribed in large enough quantities: if you have widespread eczema, a 100 g tube prescribed by your doctor is not enough. A 500 g tub should last 1–2 weeks depending on how big you are. Topical steroids should be applied in a measured way, i.e. once or twice daily as prescribed, specifically to red, inflamed areas. Most topical steroids will work well if applied only once a day so this can simplify your daily routine of applying creams.

If you have tried such a regime and things have not improved, it might be helpful to ask your doctor for a slightly greasier emollient and a topical steroid in an ointment base before wondering whether you need a stronger steroid preparation.

What do steroids do?

Steroids are essentially hormones, and there are many different types with quite different actions. The human body makes its own steroids in the adrenal gland, and these are vital for the body's normal function.

Different types of synthetic steroid have been developed for use in medicine. There is a group called anabolic steroids, which some athletes take (illegally!) to help build up muscle mass, and these should not be confused with the steroids used in eczema. The other group is called catabolic steroids or glucocorticoids (e.g. prednisolone); these are used as oral medicines in a variety of different diseases because of their anti-inflammatory and immunosuppressive properties. This means that they act by damping down the activity of various immune cells that cause inflammation.

Catabolic steroids have proved very useful in medicine, even life-saving in some medical conditions such as severe asthma and rheumatoid arthritis. The downside of this group of steroids is that if they are used in a high dose for a prolonged period, they have many side-effects, such as weight gain, bone-thinning, decreased growth in children, high blood pressure and loss of muscle mass. Because of this, doctors try to use them in the lowest possible dose for only short periods. This type of steroid is occasionally used in the treatment of a very severe flare of eczema (see Chapter 5). However, for the reasons already mentioned, it would normally be used for only a few weeks, starting at a high dose and then slowly decreasing. This method should prevent or minimise any serious side-effects.

Fortunately, these anti-inflammatory steroids can also be made into creams and ointments for topical application directly on to the skin. They act in a similar way to their oral counterparts as they have been developed to try to limit the same anti-inflammatory properties to the skin and avoid all the general (systemic) side-effects on the rest of the body, even after long-term use. This approach has been very successful, and topical steroids are one of the main components of eczema treatment.

I'm confused because my neighbour says that steroids will harm my child but the doctor says that hydrocortisone is very safe to use, even on a baby. Why is there so much conflicting information about steroids and their safety?

This is an extremely common question and concern. We are not entirely sure why so much misinformation has been generated about topical steroids, but people do seem to have extremely strong views about their safety. The anxiety about the use of topical steroids has led to a significant underuse of a very valuable form of therapy. This has caused much unnecessary suffering for children. If you talk to doctors who looked after children before the 1950s, when topical steroids were developed, you will realise what an enormous advance they have been in managing eczema.

The following points may highlight why some myths have developed:

- Some of the earliest topical steroids developed were very strong, group 1 steroids (Table 3). These readily cause thinning of the skin if used on any skin other than the palms and soles. Unfortunately, when this side-effect was first noticed, all topical steroids got a bad name because people then mistakenly thought (indeed, some still do) that the side-effects occurred even with the very weak steroids. Remember that topical steroids vary enormously in strength.

- Steroids taken by mouth have many side-effects, and many people assume that topical steroids have these too. This is untrue. Topical steroids were developed specifically to try to prevent the problems of oral steroids.

Table 3 Potencies of some topical steroids

Mild Group 4	Moderate Group 3	Potent Group 2	Very potent Group 1
Hydrocortisone 1%	Betamethasone valerate 0.025% (Betnovate-RD)	Betamethasone valerate 0.1% (Betnovate)	Clobetasol propionate 0.05% (Dermovate)
Hydrocortisone 1% + urea 10% (Calmurid HC)	Clobetasone butyrate 0.05% (Eumovate)	Betamethasone dipropionate 0.05% + salicylic acid 3% (Diprosalic)	Clobetasol propionate 0.05% + neomycin sulphate 0.5% + nystatin (Dermovate-NN)
Hydrocortisone 0.25% + crotamiton 10% (Eurax-Hydrocortisone)	Clobetasone butyrate 0.05% + oxytetracycline 3% + nystatin 100 000 units/g (Trimovate)	Fluocinolone acetonide 0.025% (Synalar N)	
Hydrocortisone 0.5% + coal tar extract 5% (Alphosyl HC)		Fluocinonide 0.05% (Metosyn)	
Hydrocortisone 1% + miconazole nitrate 2% (Daktacort)		Mometasone furoate 0.1% (Elocon)	
Hydrocortisone 1% + fusidic acid 2% (Fucidin H)		Betamethasone valerate 0.1% + fusidic acid 2% (FuciBET)	
		Hydrocortisone butyrate 0.1% + chlorquinaldol 3% (Locoid C)	

- There are different types of steroid: they act differently and have different side-effects. It is easy, though, to assume that all steroids are the same and thus misunderstand the side-effect risk. For example, anabolic steroids can cause an increase in muscle size and liver damage, but this does not occur with the topical steroids used in eczema – which are from the glucocorticoid (catabolic) group.

- Many people have become disillusioned with conventional medicine. There has been a social trend to assume that Western medicines are dangerous and that herbal remedies or natural products are safe and preferable. The word 'steroid' has become almost synonymous with all that is bad about conventional medical treatments.

- Steroids do not cure eczema, so it often recurs after using them. You may have expected a cure – partly because the media loves reporting on 'miracle cures' – and might be reluctant to use them again if there has not been one.

My doctor gave me steroid creams, but I refused to use them. Instead, I massage my body with primrose oil, which helps. What else can I do to avoid flares?

This raises a couple of issues: first, why you refused to use the steroid creams, and second, whether your present treatment is effective and, if it is not, what else could be used.

Let's tackle the difficult question first: your decision not to use topical steroids. You must ask yourself why you don't want to use them. It is often because of historical events, as described in the answer to the previous question. If, however, topical steroids are used appropriately and applied in a measured way, they can be valuable, safe and effective as part of eczema therapy. The safe use of topical steroids is paramount, but the fear of potential side-effects can often lead to underuse rather then overuse. Eczema patients often report that they find their eczema is unresponsive to steroid ointments, but the effectiveness of a treatment is often dependent on its use in conjunction with an emollient regime. Below are some guidelines for the safe use of topical steroids:

- Use topical steroids only if moisturisers and bath oils do not control the eczema, and use them only as long as is needed.

- Use topical steroids only if the eczema is red, itchy and inflamed: do not use them in place of a moisturiser on dry skin.

- Do not use topical steroids more frequently than twice daily. Note that some of the newer steroids are designed for once-daily use only, and trials of the older ones used once a day have shown that they also work at this dose.

- The strength of the topical steroid used depends upon the site of application, the extent of the eczema and your age.

- Children should always use weak group 4 steroids (see Table 3) on their face and where the skin is thinner.

- For older children, group 3/4 steroids can be used on the body. Group 2 steroids may be used for flares.

- In older children with severe eczema, group 2 steroids are occasionally used on the body. They can, however, thin the skin so they must be used for only a few days.

- With adults, group 4 steroids can be used for the face and flexures (under the arms, under the breasts and in the groin); group 3 steroids are occasionally used on these areas in flares, but medical advice must be sought. Group 3 steroids can treat eczema on the body, arms and legs, and group 2 can be used in a flare.

- Group 1 and 2 steroids are occasionally used for eczema on the palms and soles. Where the skin is thicker, however, care should be taken to avoid spread to the top of the feet or hands.

Topical steroids are effective in dealing with flares, but if you still do not feel that you could use them, maintaining an effective emollient regime will certainly be helpful to keep the skin soft and supple, and to prevent flares and irritation. The use of primrose oil will help to achieve this moisturising effect, but you should be observant over time to make sure that you do not develop a sensitivity or irritant reaction to it: that is why, in eczema management, we tend to use bland creams and ointments.

An alternative to topical steroids for controlling flares may be a topical immunomodulatory ointment called pimecrolimus. This, and another similar drug, are discussed further in the next chapter as they have not yet been established as first-line treatments for all GPs to prescribe.

My son's skin is lighter in the areas where he has had eczema – is this because of the steroid?

No, it is more likely to be because the eczema itself has caused a change in the pigmentation of the skin. The eczema can either decrease, as with your son, or increase the pigmentation. This problem can occur in anybody with eczema but is much more common in racial groups with pre-existing pigmented skin, such as those of Asian or African/Caribbean origin. This change in pigment can occur in any condition in which the skin is inflamed so can happen with other diseases such as psoriasis. Over time, the pigment should return to normal, particularly if the eczema is kept under good control.

People say that using steroids will thin my skin. This worries me as I have had eczema for years and have used steroids on and off over that time.

Be reassured that topical steroids can be used safely and the side-effects can be minimised, but only if the steroids are used appropriately, as outlined in the guidelines for steroid use earlier in this section. In addition, care must be taken in choosing the correct amounts of steroid to use, as discussed in the next question. Eczema should ideally be managed with the weakest topical steroid that will control the symptoms. Extra care should also be taken in sensitive areas such as the face, flexures (under the arms, groin, etc.) and with children. If the eczema flares, you may be advised to use a more potent steroid. Your doctor or nurse should give you accurate instructions about which steroid to use where and for how long.

If, however, very strong steroids are used on the skin for more than a few weeks, they can certainly thin the skin; this is sometimes called skin atrophy. Topical steroids are classified into four groups depending on their strength (see Table 3 on page 68). The strongest groups – 1 and 2 – are most likely to cause skin-thinning; if this happens, the skin looks thin and prematurely aged, and may wrinkle. These changes are often reversible in the early stages. With the continued application of strong topical steroids, the blood vessels in the skin become abnormally widened, or dilated, giving an appearance of stretch marks, which tends to be irreversible. There may, however, be other reasons for stretch marks developing, such as rapid growth in puberty or pregnancy.

The last time I saw the specialist, he said I needed to follow a skin-care regime and told me about the 'fingertip guide' to measuring out steroid cream, but this seems much more than I was using before – I thought I should only use it sparingly.

The term 'sparingly' is very difficult to quantify and tends to mean applying 'just enough' to the affected area: once used, a glistening layer should be seen on the skin. The 'fingertip unit' refers to a method by which you can measure the amount of topical steroid. If you squirt a line of steroid cream from the last joint in your finger to the fingertip, this equates to about an inch's worth of cream. This amount is half a gram and will treat an area of skin equivalent to the surface of the front and back of one hand. You then estimate how many fingertips of steroid you will need to treat your eczema by estimating how many 'hands-worth' of eczema you have. There are charts available to help you do this, and your nurse or doctor should be able to explain it in more detail.

The benefit of the fingertip unit is that you are using the steroid in a measured way so that correct amounts will be used without any anxiety over using too much. In addition, as an area clears, you can gradually reduce the number of 'fingertips' applied.

If this method is not used, there is a concern that you may underuse or overuse your topical steroid. It is important to follow the advice you have been given about where to use the steroid and for how long. When applying the steroid to moisturised skin, dot it over the affected area and smooth it downwards in the direction of hair growth. There is no need to massage or rub the cream into the skin.

Can steroids be used on broken skin?

'Do not use on broken skin' is often written on the packaging of topical steroid creams. This is not very helpful and is indeed rather alarmist. The nature of eczema means that there will be cracks, splits and scratches on the skin. The advice from pharmaceutical companies tends to err on the side of caution, but there is some evidence to suggest that if very large areas of broken skin are treated, increased absorption of the steroid can occur. We feel, however, that topical steroids can still be used safely, provided the correct amounts are used (as outlined in the previous question), on any patch of eczema even if it is scratched, weepy or infected – although in that case antibiotics may be needed as well. Where the skin is really broken, such as with a graze, wound or ulcer, steroids should not be used because they can delay healing.

Managing eczema in troublesome areas

The face

I have eczema on my body, but the hardest place to control it is on my face - it is so sensitive, dry and red that I have not been able to find a product to help me. What would you recommend?

The face can be a difficult area to treat. If it is very dry, the best product would ideally be grease based, but it is not always cosmetically acceptable to have a greasy face for work or school. One suggestion might be to use a grease-based moisturiser such as an emulsifying ointment or Epaderm at night or at home. These moisturisers are free from additives and preservatives, which are sometimes found in creams and can cause sensitivity reactions. In addition, the same ointment could be used as a soap substitute to cleanse the face.

When the skin becomes inflamed and very dry, you may often find that whatever you use seems to sting a little at first; this can sometimes be reduced by a soap-substitute wash followed directly by the application of a moisturiser. It is worth remembering that when a moisturiser is applied, the affected areas appear more obvious and red for a short time afterwards. If a cream is preferred for daytime use, try to use a greasy cream (see Table 2 on page 64); you could try a test area first to check your tolerance of this. This regime could be used in conjunction with a topical steroid, but if the problem persists on your face, it may be helpful to see a specialist to rule out the possibility of contact sensitivity to any of the ingredients in the creams you are using.

My eczema has been erupting on my lips and in the corners of my mouth, as well as around my nostrils. It is very painful, cracked, bleeding and itchy. This is very unattractive and embarrassing. What can I do?

If these areas are cracking, there is a need for increased moisturising. When the skin becomes very dry, it loses its usual flexibility and suppleness, and as a consequence the skin cracks and splits. So frequently using a grease-based moisturiser on these areas will be helpful. It will be helpful to decant some moisturiser into a small container so that it is easily accessible during the day.

The other aspect to consider is whether anything in this area is causing an irritation – for example, toothpaste while brushing the teeth, or soap when cleansing the face.

Finally, if these cracks persist, it may be helpful to use a topical steroid on these areas, sometimes in combination with either an antibacterial or antifungal agent. You can discuss this further with your own doctor.

I have persistent eczema around the eye area, and my GP has suggested moisturising and hydrocortisone cream. Can you suggest any type of cream more suited to this sensitive area?

The area around the eyes can be difficult to treat, for a couple of reasons. It is very sensitive so only the weakest steroids should be used. It is also possible for creams applied in this area to be absorbed or accidentally rubbed into the eyes – if this happens regularly over weeks or months, it can lead to the development of cataracts or increased pressure in the eyes, called glaucoma. Your GP's suggestion sounds very good and safe, especially if you use the moisturiser regularly, combine it with a soap substitute and limit your use of the hydrocortisone (a weak steroid) to a few days at a time to settle any flares.

If you do not respond to this, we would recommend referral to see whether you have any allergies causing the eczema around your eyes. If you do, you may be able to stop the eczema by avoiding certain creams and make-up. If not, the consultant might try you on one of the new immunomodulatory creams such as pimecrolimus or tacrolimus. These have none of the skin-thinning side-effects seen with the overuse of steroids and do not cause any problems by being used close to the eyes. They can, however, be irritant in the first few days of use. This usually wears off but may be troublesome on the face.

Recently, my outer ears became itchy, and now just inside my ears is scaly and crusty. I wonder whether eczema is a danger to my hearing.

No, eczema is not a danger to your hearing. However, as you describe, eczema can certainly affect the ear canal as it is just a rolled-up tube of skin. If the ear canal is dry and scaly, you may find that the scale will bind with the usual earwax and cause some blockage of the canal. This can be treated simply with warm olive oil, which will soften the scale. If the ear canal is red and inflamed, you may find it helpful to use some steroid eardrops to reduce irritation.

For the past year, I have been prescribed Modrasone cream for my eczema, which appears as hot, red pimples with white heads around the lower area of my face. The cream soothes the inflammation after a day or so, but as soon as one area starts to clear up, another outbreak occurs close by. Is there anything else I can do as I feel the cream is becoming less effective?

We would advise that you revisit your doctor for a review. Topical steroids come in different strengths, and Modrasone is a group 3 steroid (see Table 3 on page 68), which means that it is of moderate strength. A year is a long time to use a steroid such as this on your face as the facial skin is delicate and more prone to developing some of the potential side-effects of topical steroids.

You describe your skin as having red pimples with white heads – it sounds as if you have developed a different condition called perioral dermatitis, which creates spots (as in acne), inflammation and itching. It is caused by using a more potent steroid on the face and is treated with a course of antibiotics, which we commonly use in acne. If this is the case, you need to stop the topical steroid and allow the skin to settle. When you do this, the skin often becomes worse before it gets better so we sometimes suggest weaning off the stronger steroid to a weaker one, such as hydrocortisone, at the same time as starting the course of antibiotics.

The genital area

Can you recommend a treatment for chronic genital eczema; I am so depressed with it.

It might be helpful to review your whole regime of treatment. Are you avoiding all irritants like soaps and detergents, and remembering to use a soap substitute such as aqueous cream or emulsifying ointment? Generally speaking, a bath is more beneficial than a shower. If you are able to have a bath, ask your doctor for a bath oil to soften the water and ease the irritation. In addition, find a moisturiser that you are comfortable with – the greasier the better – and reapply it after every time you go to the toilet.

Have you used a topical steroid on this area and, if so, was it a cream or an ointment? Ointments are generally more effective in this area, and using a combination of an antibacterial and an antifungal agent can be helpful here too. If the irritation persists, it might be helpful for your doctor to swab the area to ensure there is no yeast infection (such as thrush). It is also helpful to consider whether anything else may be making this problem worse: for example, do you use condoms, pessaries or any other creams or gels on this area, which might be causing the irritation?

We give patients the following handout with advice for minimising itching 'down below':

- Avoid using any soaps and deodorants on the vulval area.

- Use a soap substitute – it can be stored in the fridge as this makes it much more soothing. Use it to cleanse the area before getting into the bath or shower.

- Stop all bubble baths.

- Do not shampoo your hair in the bath.

- Never use antiseptics such as Dettol or TCP in the bath.

- Avoid rubbing the area with a flannel; use cotton wool, your fingertips or a soft cloth.

- Dry your skin thoroughly after a bath or shower – you can even use a cool hairdryer to avoid rubbing the skin with a towel.

- If it is convenient, wear a loose skirt without underwear for some time each day.

- Avoid tight clothes, especially if they are made of synthetic material, as they reduce ventilation and increase humidity in this area.

- Avoid tights – stockings are better. Always wear cotton underwear.

- Do not use talcum powder as it tends to collect in crevices; even baby powder should be avoided.

- Scratching should be avoided at all costs as it can further damage the skin. If this is a problem at night, wear light cotton gloves and keep your nails short. If the irritation is unbearable, pinching is preferable to scratching as it is less likely to break the skin surface.

The feet and hands

I have severe eczema affecting my feet. I've tried steroid cream and moisturisers, but this brings little effect. Is there anything else you could suggest?

It might be helpful to use an intensive treatment for a short time. Use lots of greasy moisturiser on the feet and wrap some cling-film around them, leaving it on overnight. You will find that this will have a softening effect on thick, dry skin, especially if you can repeat the treatment each night for about a week. It is a very effective way to rehydrate such very dry, thickened skin and make it much easier for a strong steroid cream, applied in the morning, to penetrate the skin. You can occasionally use the same technique with steroid and emollient, but this should only be done with medical advice as the occlusion caused by the cling-film will cause the steroid to be absorbed even more readily, giving a greater chance of local side-effects in the skin.

I have started to suffer from warped and cracked thumbnails. When they are particularly bad, they become increasingly painful – the slightest knock creates searing pain, and raw skin is exposed through the crack in the nail. Can I stop this happening?

It may be helpful for you to see your doctor or a specialist first to confirm that eczema is the cause of these nail problems. Eczema can affect the nails to a varying degree, and if eczema is confirmed, a couple of approaches will help.

First, a steroid cream or ointment can be rubbed specifically into the cracked areas of the nails. Alternatively, your doctor could prescribe a steroid scalp application, which can be drizzled down under the affected part of the nail more effectively. Keeping the nails well trimmed can help, and wrapping tape (such as Micropore) around the nail and fingertip can be useful to prevent trauma to the nail. If the nail is intact with no sign of active eczema, false nails can be used to cover any abnormalities as long as the adhesive does not cause any irritation of the surrounding skin.

Second, it helps to follow a good hand-care regime, as described below:

- Avoid soaps and detergents. Use a soap substitute, and wear protective gloves (preferably latex-free) when dealing with detergents.

- Avoid handling or preparing irritant foods such as citrus fruits, onions, chillies, raw vegetables (especially tomatoes) and salty food.

- Use moisturisers frequently during the day.

- Wear cotton gloves for 'dry' jobs in the home or garden.

The scalp

My eczema is on the back of my neck and in my hair. I have tried all sorts of shampoos and creams but find it is spreading down my neck so that other people notice the eczema when I wear my hair up. Are there any better treatments I could use?

The scalp can be a fiddly area to treat, and the best results are often seen when someone else is able to treat your scalp for you. When you treat yourself, you are relying on touch rather than vision to find the affected areas, and much of the treatment lands in the hair rather than on the scalp.

Scalp eczema tends to respond well to a scalp application of topical steroid. If you have tried one of these already, it is worth checking whether it was in an alcohol or an aqueous base. The clear liquids tend to contain alcohol, which can sting and burn, whereas the lotion is water based and can have a calmer, more moisturising effect on the scalp. A mousse preparation is also available, which you could try as an alternative.

To cleanse your hair, use simple baby shampoo or a mild medicated shampoo. Tar shampoos can also be of help, but some people find tar irritant and drying so caution should be exercised to make sure that it will not make things worse. If your neck and hair line are also affected, it can be useful to rub a greasy, water-based moisturiser into these areas and leave it overnight. In the morning, cleanse and apply more moisturiser and steroid.

I have recently developed scalp eczema and have lost my hair in the process. Can you tell me why this has happened, and will my hair grow back?

When there is a lot of scaling and inflammation of the scalp, the hair shafts can break and split. The consequence is that hair will be lost as scale lifts from the scalp. In this type of hair loss, the hair will regrow and settle once the eczema is under better control. Care must be taken to use grease and oils to soften the scale effectively before it is lifted from the scalp as if scale is lifted when dry and attached firmly to the hair and scalp, it will tend to cause trauma to the base and may damage the hair follicles.

There are other conditions that cause hair loss, such as alopecia areata so, if you have regained control of the eczema but the hair loss is persisting, it is worth seeking advice from your doctor to confirm what else could be causing it.

Chronic eczema – approaches to therapy

You might find that, despite trying hard to avoid things that make your eczema worse and despite a regular treatment regime, your eczema still persists. The itching, rubbing and scratching of the skin can occasionally cause the skin to become dry and thickened; this change in skin is known as lichenification.

This section covers some other treatments that can help. They should be regarded as extra treatments to be added to the topical therapies previously mentioned.

My son scratches a lot at night and wakes up every morning with blood on his sheets. He seems much less itchy in the day. Why is this?

Itching is often worse at night, and there could be a number of reasons for this:

- It is warmer at night because of being covered by bedding, and an increase in temperature increases feelings of itchiness.

- There are not so many distractions at night as there are during the day so once the itching starts at night it is easy to focus solely on that, and a non-stop itch–scratch cycle can develop.

- Finally, the presence of house dust mite in bedding and on soft toys (see later in this chapter) may be important in making the eczema worse in some children.

I cannot sleep at night because of the pain and itching. I am at my wits' end so what should I be asking my GP to do?

If we assume that you are using emollients and topical steroids as well as you can, you may need to add something to block out the itch and help you sleep. Because eczema is sometimes caused by allergies and is linked to asthma and hay fever, antihistamine tablets are often tried. The non-sedative ones that are useful for hay fever do not seem to work very well, with the possible exception of one called fexofenadine, so the older, more sedative types are used. It may be the sedation rather than the antihistamine effect that works, but whatever it is, it can help you to sleep and break the cycle of scratching all night. The other thing to consider is bandaging the skin over a layer of emollient.

There are a lot of bedding products on the market at the moment. Can you tell me which is the best one to use?

There are indeed a large number of bedding products, and we need to explain about house dust mite to understand this approach to treatment. The house dust mite is a microscopic organism, invisible to the naked eye, that loves living in soft furnishings. It can undoubtedly make asthma worse, but evidence about its role in provoking atopic eczema is still limited. It is in fact the house dust mite droppings that cause an allergic response by bringing enzymes from the mite's gut into contact with the skin.

Some bedding products aim to reduce the number of house dust mites coming into contact with your skin, but none will eradicate it all together. They may be divided into two groups:

Mattress covers. Several mattress covers are claimed to decrease the number of house dust mites in bedding. A recent trial using Gortex mattress, duvet and pillow covers, in combination with regular damp-dusting and vacuuming, showed an improvement in some individuals with atopic eczema, but Gortex is unfortunately no longer marketed in the UK for mattress covers. Other trials of bedding covers have been less convincing. They all lead to a decrease in the number of house dust mites, but this does not always benefit atopic eczema sufferers.

Bedding sprays. There are a number of spray products, called acaricides, on the market, aimed at killing mites in bedding. They have a variety of chemical names, such as natamycin, benzyl benzoate, tannic acid, benzyl tannate and bioallethrin. All produce a variable decrease in the number of house dust mites, but when used in isolation they rarely have a significant effect on atopic eczema. This may be because they do not get rid of the house dust mite droppings so repeated washing of the bedding is also needed.

Unfortunately, no study has compared the treatment options mentioned above so we do not know whether one is better than another. There are also other factors to consider in the house dust mite story. The following tend to increase the number of house dust mites:

- late summer;
- hot, humid conditions;
- older houses;
- older mattresses.

The 'reducing house dust mite' approach requires a lot of effort and has significant cost implications – these products are not available on prescription. The sprays need to be repeated, every 6–12 weeks, and the covers regularly replaced, every 6–12 months. Using one option in isolation tends not to work. A combination of covers, sprays and vacuuming/damp-dusting is more likely to be effective but is no guarantee of success. On balance, we feel that for such a relatively small improvement in atopic eczema, we would not recommend this costly approach as a routine first-line treatment. If atopic eczema is proving to be very severe and unresponsive to treatment, and you also have asthma, the approach may be worth a trial for 2–3 months, provided the family is feeling very motivated.

More clinical trials are needed to compare the effectiveness of the different sprays and covers in improving atopic eczema rather than just in their ability to remove house dust mites.

Information on the manufacturers of bedding products can be obtained from the National Eczema Society (see Appendix 1).

Can you recommend a vacuum cleaner that will get rid of house dust mites?

Most vacuum cleaners reduce to some degree the number of house dust mites in carpets, but they will certainly not eradicate them. Modern vacuum cleaners with filters may decrease dust mites more efficiently, but a recent study suggested that there is little to choose between the different makes of vacuum cleaner when it comes to improving eczema. In an ideal world, it would be better to get rid of carpets and replace them with linoleum, tiled or wood floors. These can be regularly damp-dusted or washed.

Bear in mind, however, that carpets are not the only good home for house dust mites. All soft furnishings, including sofas, mattresses, duvets, etc., harbour house dust mites, and it is worth taking soft cuddly toys into account if you are having a real 'blitz'. In fact, bedding harbours more mites than carpets do. Therefore, vacuuming alone is unlikely to have a significant impact on the house dust mite population. Although house dust mites may be important in causing asthma, we still do not know how important they are in atopic eczema.

My baby developed eczema at the age of 4 months. She is now 6 months old, and on the whole her eczema is under control with topical treatments from the GP. However, her face is always very red and sore, particularly when she wakes up in the morning, despite using moisturisers last thing at night. What should I do?

It might be worth thinking about the cot and bedding material. With a new baby, well-meaning relatives often offer you the cots, prams, etc. that they no longer require. If this is the case, the house dust mite content of a second-hand mattress will be exceptionally high and irritate your baby's face. If possible, invest in a new mattress and/or a mattress cover.

Always ensure that mittens are worn at night to limit scratching and that the sheets are soft cotton or silk as it is not uncommon for babies to rub their faces on bedding if they cannot scratch. There are other general measures to consider, too:

- Vacuum the mattress thoroughly at least once a week.

- Never use feather pillows or duvets.

- Try to use a foam mattress or, if this is not possible, use a mattress cover.

- Don't put toys, books or any other items that may collect dust on shelves above the bed.

My son seems to have become resistant to the Vallergan I give him at night.

This quite commonly occurs if one particular antihistamine is used regularly every night: children seem to become tolerant to the effect of the drug. This can sometimes be prevented by using the Vallergan (alimemazine, formerly known as trimeprazine) intermittently, keeping it for times when the eczema is flaring. An alternative strategy would be to change to a different antihistamine, such as hydroxyzine (Atarax), promethazine (Phenergan) or chlorphenamine (Piriton).

Very rarely, antihistamines seem to make children hyperactive rather than sleepy. This does not mean that the other antihistamines will do the same, so changing over is the best option.

Bandaging

My elderly mother has had dry itchy eczema on her legs for some months, and we have tried various creams. The GP has now suggested we see the nurse for extra help and advice. He said we may need to use paste bandages – what are they?

Paste bandages can be useful in treating eczema where the skin has become thickened (lichenified) as a response to repeated scratching, or where there are multiple cracks and scratches (excoriations). Paste bandages can be very beneficial for this type of eczema in the short term, as they:

- allow scratched areas to heal;
- let the creams work more effectively by increasing their absorption;
- prevent further damage to the skin and help to break the itch–scratch cycle.

- provide a constant environment for the skin, avoiding changes in the temperature and humidity of the skin, which helps to lessen the itch; changes in temperature such as getting undressed or getting out of a warm bath often make people feel itchy even if they do not have eczema.

It sounds as if your mother has persevered with her treatment regime but needs a slightly more intensive treatment for a while. A number of paste bandages are available on prescription; we commonly use either zinc oxide bandages, such as Viscopaste, Steripaste or Zipzoc, or ichthammol bandages, such as Ichthopaste or Ichthaband. The choice depends on the appearance of the eczema.

Using a paste bandage is just one step on from topical therapy. It consists of the following stages:

- Wash using a bath emollient/soap substitute (you might find the nurse soaks your mother's leg in a bucket – the floor-washing type is the best shape).

- Apply generous amounts of emollient/moisturiser to all areas.

- Apply topical steroid only to the affected areas.

- Apply paste bandage to the affected areas (see the question below).

- Apply the top retaining bandage (e.g. K-band) and stockinette (e.g. Tubifast) to hold the paste bandage in place. An adhesive bandage such as Coban is occasionally used to retain the paste bandage; this is particularly helpful in children and the elderly to prevent premature removal of the bandage.

Paste bandages can be left in place for 2–3 days, after which they begin to become very dry and irritating. You mention that your mother is going to see the nurse; she will probably need to visit three times a week to have the bandages applied. However, the bandaging is something that the nurse could teach you to do for your mother at home, if you felt able to take it on.

We use paste bandages for my daughter's eczema. They are very effective, but we were wondering why we have to put them on in pleats. Is there an easier way to use them?

Yes, paste bandages can work well but are sometimes a fiddle to apply – well done for working with them as it sounds like you have had some pleasing results. Below are some points to explain the application notes for paste bandages:

- The paste bandage is a wet bandage and should *not* be applied to limbs in a round-and-round, spiral fashion (i.e. the way in which a crêpe bandage is applied to a sprained ankle). It should be applied either in strips wrapped round the limb or in a forwards-and-backwards pleating action – it is always best that someone demonstrates this to you.

- This technique allows for any drying or shrinkage of the bandage, which might cause constriction of the limb and damage to the blood supply.

- Once you are used to applying the paste bandages, they can be used in a more flexible way, such as patches over small troublesome areas or night-time use only.

- Zipzoc is a tubular zinc paste bandage that can be slipped over the limb; this can sometimes be helpful for eczema sufferers who are self-treating.

All the bandages mentioned here can be prescribed by your doctor or nurse. It is important to get the right number of bandages so that you have enough to continue the treatment over a few weeks.

My friend also has eczema. She has been using wet-wrap bandages and I would like to try them, but I am not sure how they work or whether my GP will prescribe them. Are they the same as paste bandages?

Wet-wrapping is a special bandaging technique that can be used to treat all areas of skin, including the face. This was traditionally a treatment carried out in hospital, but it has more recently been used in the home environment.

The wet-wrap technique involves using two layers of a tubi-stockinette bandage (e.g. Tubifast, Comfifast), which are cut to fit the affected area. Emollients are applied liberally to all areas and the topical steroid as prescribed to the affected areas only. The inner layer of stockinette is soaked in warm water – hence the name wet-wraps – and then the top layer is applied dry. Over time, the bandage will dry out so, during the day, the outer layer can be pulled down and the inner layer remoistened with warm water: a clean plant-sprayer can be used to do this quickly and effectively. Then the top dry layer is replaced.

Whole body wet-wraps can be used for severe widespread eczema, i.e. when the skin is red and inflamed, which is called erythrodermic eczema and can cause the individual to feel unwell. Fortunately, this is very rare and is best managed in the hospital setting.

In the home setting, however, wet-wraps can be used after specific education and support. They can be used on specific troublesome areas such as arms and legs and do not have to be applied to the whole body. If the eczema is widespread, stockinette garments can be prescribed for children, or varying sizes of stockinette to treat an adult. The wet-wraps are a useful way to control inflamed eczema, but the wet-wrapping causes increased absorption of the steroid and can only be used for short periods of time – 3–7 days. In addition, wet-wrapping should be avoided in infected eczema, owing to the warm, moist environment, which will provide ideal conditions for the growth of bacteria.

Wet-wraps can also be used over emollients, without any steroid, for exceptionally dry eczema; however, a single dry layer of stockinette over emollients can often be just as effective and is easier to apply. So we would advise that this is a useful first step before embarking on wet-wrapping.

Psychological aspects

I seem to scratch constantly with my eczema. Sometimes my partner tells me to stop scratching, but I don't even know that I am doing it. When I start to scratch, it just seems impossible to stop. What can I do?

Be reassured that you are not alone. When you have had eczema for some time, it is possible to get stuck in an itch–scratch cycle. This can become habitual, and at times you may be scratching even though you are not aware of an itchy sensation. The itching and scratching can become totally absorbing, and some patients with eczema describe a sensation of pleasure from scratching itchy skin; others feel they cannot stop scratching until the skin bleeds. A lot of research has been carried out among dermatologists, nurses and psychiatrists at the Chelsea and Westminster Hospital, London, who have devised techniques to break the itch–scratch cycle called 'habit reversal'.

First, your eczema treatment needs to be optimised. Write a list of irritants, emollients, bathing products, topical steroids, infections, antihistamines and bandages. Consider each point in turn and see how it is being handled. Can anything be improved? Consider whether you have a different regime for flares and for maintenance treatment. Discuss any worries with your GP or nurse. It is sometimes helpful to develop a new approach and aim to take control of the eczema. Manage, don't *be* managed!

The next step of habit reversal usually involves a session with a psychologist, doctor or nurse. They often advise using a hand-held counter during the first week to record how much scratching is occurring. This raises your awareness of when you scratch and you can highlight situations when scratching is worse. Having a greater awareness of scratching allows you to develop techniques to avoid further scratching, such as:

- clenching your fists and counting to 30;
- pinching or pressing on the skin rather than scratching;
- keeping creams in the fridge and applying these cold creams instead of scratching;

- being aware that changes in temperature can trigger an itchy sensation so having clothes and creams at the ready when bathing and changing;

- trying other methods of distraction – television, reading, music or relaxation techniques.

Tell other members of the family that you are trying to tackle this difficult problem. It is best if they don't shout 'Stop scratching!' as it is rather demoralising, but they could remind you of something distracting to do.

Regular follow-up and support will help you get through this. Remember that this approach is helpful but is just one aspect of treatment and should be used in conjunction with other therapies.

Scarring

Are there cures for the scars that I have from my eczema. They are dark brown; I don't know if this is what they call pigmentation. Is there something I should use on them?

After the inflammation has settled following a flare of eczema, you can sometimes be left with 'post-inflammatory hyperpigmentation'. This can last a number of months or even years but will gradually fade over time.

How can I get rid of the marks from eczema?

Continue to use a regular moisturiser on the area. If there is active eczema, treat this with a topical steroid. Generally speaking, scars from excoriations are unlikely. Even when someone seems to gouge out pieces of skin, it is amazing how well the skin recovers its normal state once the eczema has improved. Darker patches can sometimes develop with pigmented skin, as described above.

5
Second-line treatment of eczema

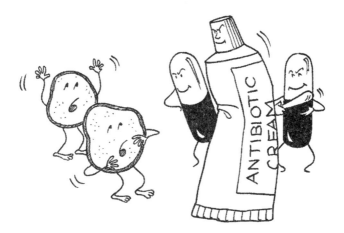

Introduction

This chapter discusses further treatments and is divided into four sections, dealing with:

- infection;
- treatment in hospital;
- phototherapy (ultraviolet light treatment);
- treatment taken by mouth.

Although infection is a relatively common complication of atopic eczema, the treatments discussed in the other sections of this chapter are relevant to only a small number of people because they are reserved for very severe disease. Severity must, of course, be regarded from the person's own perspective rather than from that of the doctor.

The appearance and extent of the eczema are not all that should be considered as the effect on quality of life is just as important. This can be especially important for children, for whom growth suppression, time off school, severe disruption of sleep (which can affect the whole family) and difficulties fitting into friendship groups at school are some of the most important factors to be considered when judging severity. Similar issues apply to adults, especially when the ability to work can seriously affect someone's finances. It often does not matter what underlying cause or type of eczema you have; the principles of what is often called 'second-line treatment' remain much the same.

Coping with infection

I think my eczema might be infected. Should I still use the steroid cream?

Yes, you should, but you will also need to treat the infection. If it is very localised, treatment can be with an antibiotic cream or a combination of steroid and antibiotic in the same tube. Infection is often, however, more widespread so antibiotics by mouth are more appropriate.

Bacterial infection can be caused by either staphylococci or streptococci – two different types of bacterium. The former is much more common, accounting for 90% of cases, and responds well to an antibiotic called flucloxacillin, usually given for 7–10 days. Penicillin V is used for streptococci. Erythromycin and similar antibiotics can be used in either case if you are allergic to penicillin-type antibiotics.

My eczema is very wet. What is the best way to treat it?

Wet or weepy eczema may be infected so you may well need a course of antibiotics. The wetness is also a sign that the eczema is very acute and inflamed, so topical steroids are needed as well, but, as discussed in the section on 'Moisturisers and emollients' in Chapter 4, a cream formulation should be used as ointments tend to 'float off' very wet eczema and do not get absorbed into the skin.

If the eczema on your hands is very weepy, it can be worth using soaks made up of potassium permanganate to dry it out quickly. This is available as crystals or tablets (Permitabs), which are dissolved in water to give a dark purple solution. This should be diluted with more water until it is a light pink colour before use as strong solutions will stain the skin and nails brown and can cause skin irritation. The hands should be soaked for 20 minutes at a time, twice a day. There are two different ways of using the solution:

- The first is by simply immersing the hands in the solution.

- The second is by soaking gauze squares or an old flannel and laying this over the eczema. This technique allows other areas to be treated as well if they cannot be immersed.

The potassium permanganate solution is antiseptic and also very drying so should be used only for 2 or 3 days. If you use too strong a solution and notice some brown staining of your nails, don't worry – it will not be permanent!

I keep getting bouts of infection and am very worried about all the antibiotics I have to take. Are there any other treatments I could use?

Yes, there are some alternatives. One approach is to try a topical antibiotic as a cream or ointment. This can be used as soon as any sign of infection develops but is only really suitable for quite localised areas.

There are a number of combination preparations containing a topical steroid in different strengths with an antibiotic. Weak (group 4; see Table 3 on page 68) steroid combinations include Vioform-Hydrocortisone (clioquinol and hydrocortisone) and Fucidin H (fusidic acid and hydrocortisone) cream. These are suitable for use anywhere because the steroid is of low potency. Betnovate-C (betamethasone and clioquinol), Locoid C (hydrocortisone butyrate and chlorquinaldol) and FuciBET (betamethasone and fusidic acid) all contain strong (group 2) steroids and should only be used for short periods, avoiding the face and flexures if possible. Wet, infected eczema allows creams to penetrate more easily into the skin so even more care is needed with the stronger steroids.

Although the above can help, even topical antibiotics can cause bacterial resistance to develop, and it is important to keep their use to a minimum. It can be a good idea to use separate tubes of antibiotic and steroids to avoid the temptation of using the antibiotic/steroid combination for longer than the antibiotic is needed, which will cause resistance problems. Another approach is to use antiseptics. These come in a variety of different forms, mainly as bath oil preparations such as Oilatum Plus (liquid paraffin, benzalkonium and triclosan), or Emulsiderm and Dermol 600 (liquid paraffin, isopropyl myristate and benzalkonium), or as moisturisers/soap substitutes such as Dermol 500 (liquid paraffin, benzalkonium, chlorhexidine and isopropyl myristate) or Dermol 200, which is just the same but packaged in a shower gel-type container. You should use these as a long-term preventive measure to reduce the number of bacteria on your skin. It is best to avoid commercial antiseptic soaps as the detergent content can make the eczema worse.

If you still get recurrent bouts of infection, it can be worth having swabs taken from inside your nose to see whether you are harbouring the bacteria there. If so, you can use mupirocin – an antibiotic in a special cream designed for use in the nostrils.

My daughter developed eczema herpeticum last year and was successfully treated for it. She is due to start school next month, and I know that it is likely that she will come into contact with children with cold sores. Is it possible for her to become infected with eczema herpeticum again? If so, can I do anything to reduce the risks?

Eczema herpeticum is a rare but serious complication of eczema. Fortunately, it usually occurs only once, although a small proportion of children do suffer from recurrent attacks. Each episode can, however, be treated in the same way, with a 5-day course of antiviral tablets or liquid taken by mouth. As you will be much more aware of the problems it can cause, you are much more likely to spot any sign of recurrence quickly and get the treatment started before it becomes serious.

In general, cold sores are more common in adults than in children, but there still is some chance of exposure at school. In practice, it is difficult to prevent exposure to the herpes virus completely because it is so widespread, so if someone does have an active cold sore your daughter should avoid close contact as spread only happens with touching. Doting relatives should avoid kissing her if they have an active cold sore, and you should be able to explain this to them diplomatically! School can be more difficult as refusing to sit next to someone with a cold sore may be met by the retaliation of refusing to sit next to someone with eczema! This should be discussed with the teacher so that any possible problems are handled delicately. Once again, it is worth explaining that as long as eczema herpeticum is quickly recognised and treated, it is not dangerous.

How do you treat molluscum contagiosum?

Molluscum contagiosum is a viral infection that resolves spontaneously with no treatment, although this can take, on average, up to 12 months. The individual lesions can be treated by freezing them with liquid nitrogen, but this is very cold so can be painful and is only tolerated by older children and adults. Liquid nitrogen also needs to be used with care if the skin is pigmented as it can affect the colour and leave a white patch, which is permanent.

Old-fashioned treatments include squeezing the lesions with forceps or pricking in some phenol with a needle. We feel that these treatments are painful and can sometimes cause scarring so are best avoided. In most cases, the best policy is to leave well alone so we would consider treatment only if they were visible and causing distress.

Treatment in hospital

My eczema wasn't responding to good treatment from my GP so I went to see a consultant. She prescribed a different cream called tacrolimus, which seems to be working. Why couldn't my GP give me this one?

Tacrolimus and a related cream, called pimecrolimus, are relatively new. In fact, they are the first really new forms of treatment for eczema since steroids came along in the 1950s. They are referred to as 'calcineurin inhibitors'. Calcineurin is an enzyme in the skin that plays an important part in the process of inflammation, which leads to obvious eczema. Steroids also block this process but only very bluntly, which leads to their side-effects on other structures in the skin. It is known that the two new drugs are free from the side-effects of skin-thinning and stretch marks that are associated with steroids, but we still need to be cautious about their safety in the long term. There are some concerns about an increased risk of skin cancer if they are used for long periods of time. For these reasons, it is recommended that they are only used by GPs with a particular interest and experience in treating eczema and by consultant dermatologists.

These medications are also licensed for use only in atopic eczema so if you do not have this type of eczema, your GP has more reason not to use them. Many treatments in medicine are used on conditions for which they are not licensed, but this occurs where there is a lot of experience of their use and evidence that they work and are safe. This evidence tends to start from consultant use and spread out to GPs once it has been accepted as 'common practice'. If your consultant decides that this is a good cream for you to use, your GP might well agree to prescribe it in the future.

Is tacrolimus better than steroids?

No, it seems to be equivalent to a potent topical steroid such as betamethasone (found in Betnovate) but is more expensive. As the risk of using steroids wrongly is well known and can be avoided by correct use – in the short term and as weak as will do the job – they are still regarded as the first-line treatment. Tacrolimus is reserved for cases that seem to be resistant to steroids or when there have already been side-effects from excessive steroid use in the past. It may become more used on vulnerable sites such as the face and flexures as it becomes more established and we all become more familiar with its use.

Is pimecrolimus also as good as a potent steroid?

No, it seems to be different from tacrolimus, and its place in the choices to treat eczema is less clear. More research is being carried out and may clarify this issue in the future. Pimecrolimus has been positioned by its manufacturers as a treatment to be used as soon as your skin starts to flare so it could fit in between using moisturisers alone and adding in a weak steroid like hydrocortisone. Its strength seems to be much more like that of hydrocortisone, and some people feel that using a little bit of hydrocortisone may be just as good and as safe for early flares. Once again, pimecrolimus is free from the potential side-effects of steroids and may be suitable for some patients.

My 4-year-old son has very severe eczema but has been improving with tacrolimus ointment from the hospital. Can I be sure that it is a safe treatment for him – he is using an 'adult strength'?

Tacrolimus is quite new so has been through a very rigorous testing procedure. It comes in two strengths – one for children (0.03%) and one for adults (0.1%) – but many consultants are using the stronger one in young children, with no reported major problems.

Like all active drugs, tacrolimus can have some side-effects, the main problem being some burning and tingling in the first few days of use. This usually settles and can be eased by using a mild steroid for a few days as well. What we do not yet know is its long-term safety if patients have to use it for prolonged and repeated courses. This will apply to only a few severe cases as, like steroids, it should only need to be used for short courses in the majority of people.

Tacrolimus has an effect on the immune system in the skin so there are concerns about whether this might affect the skin's ability to repair damage from ultraviolet light and lead to an increased risk of skin cancer in the future. It is sensible to make sure that your son is well protected from the sun to counteract this potential increased risk. As this is a long-term concern, we will probably not have an answer, one way or the other, for many years.

Can children using tacrolimus have the usual immunisations?

Yes, they can. This has also been looked at because the ointment has an effect on immune processes in the skin. The only advice is to avoid giving the injection through a patch of skin where tacrolimus is being used. The same advice applies to pimecrolimus.

I am doing well with tacrolimus but have recently noticed that my face goes red when I have an alcoholic drink. This never used to happen – could there be some connection?

Yes, as the list of potential side-effects includes a warning about alcohol 'intolerance', which seems to cause facial flushing in some cases. It is probably sensible to avoid alcohol when using the ointment, but you should have no problems in between courses.

Another possible answer is that you have developed a condition called rosacea, which causes little red bumps and spots over the cheeks and nose. It can be associated with flushing with alcohol or spicy foods. It might be worth double-checking your diagnosis with your doctor if you think that this is a possibility.

My son has bad eczema and has been admitted to hospital twice for treatment. He gets better quickly despite using therapy similar to the one I use at home. Why is this?

The treatment you use at home probably consists of moisturisers, bath oils and topical steroid creams. Although your hospital may have used similar therapy, there are many other differences between the hospital and home environments. Eczema is a 'multifactorial' condition – many different factors are involved in triggering it, keeping it going and making it worse. There may be several reasons why your son responds differently in hospital, and these can also apply to adults who just need a break from the daily grind of applying creams:

- Children often benefit from a change of environment and a fresh approach to their skin, which can have important psychological benefits.

- Children may feel more relaxed, especially if families have developed high levels of stress from their disrupted sleep patterns and constant scratching. In addition, playing with the nurses and other children on the ward may provide regular distraction from scratching. Parents may also feel relieved and more relaxed after a break from routine, monotonous skin-care regimes: children are very sensitive to parental anxiety.

- Concordance with treatment is usually very high during inpatient treatment even if children are usually rather reluctant and uncooperative.

- Hospital wards have very little in the way of soft furnishings and therefore have a lower level of house dust mite than is usually found at home.

Inpatient therapy is a useful option when eczema has become very severe. It does not mean that anybody has failed. Instead, it provides an opportunity to improve the eczema rapidly, to develop a fresh approach and to give both the child and the parents a well-earned break from all the monotony and hard work.

Phototherapy (ultraviolet light treatment)

I have heard that sunshine helps eczema. Will using a sunbed help my skin?

To answer this, we first need to explain about ultraviolet light and sunshine. Natural sunlight consists of two ultraviolet wavelengths, called UVA and UVB.

UVB may help to improve inflammatory skin conditions such as eczema. Artificial UVB is occasionally used to treat eczema but only if the eczema is severe and not responding well to standard first-line therapy (see Chapter 4). UVB treatment is carried out only in hospital dermatology departments, where doses are strictly controlled. It is given three times a week over a 6–10-week course. Special goggles must be worn during treatment to protect the eyes.

UVA therapy alone is not very effective at treating skin disorders. When it is used to treat eczema, it has to be given with a photosensitising medicine, called a psoralen, to make the UVA work more effectively. This psoralen can be given by mouth or applied to the skin in the bath water. This treatment is called PUVA therapy: **p**soralen + **UVA**. It is given only twice a week, but the sunglasses must be worn during the whole of the day of treatment because the psoralen will continue to sensitise the eyes even to natural sunshine.

Both UVB and PUVA treatment can irritate eczema at the start of treatment. Therefore, to begin with, they are given at very low doses, occasionally with oral steroid 'cover'. The dose is then slowly built up during the course of the treatment. Because these are specialist treatments, they must be carefully monitored.

To return to your question about sunbed usage, most sunbeds are aimed at tanning the skin and consist of predominantly UVA light – so they are not very effective in treating eczema. Moreover, because the doses are not measured adequately, they can do more harm than good.

Both UVB and PUVA can cause skin damage, and even skin cancer, later in life if *too much* is given. PUVA carries a higher risk than UVB so its use is more restricted. For safety, there is a maximum number of PUVA treatments allowed over a lifetime (about 10 courses). The risk of skin damage is much lower for people with an Asian or African/Caribbean skin type. Those with pale skin, blue eyes, red hair and freckles are most at risk so we would not usually recommend phototherapy in this group.

Phototherapy is certainly useful for severe eczema but can be inconvenient, even though the treatment takes only a few minutes each time, because it entails several visits to a hospital department. However, most departments have early-morning or late-evening appointments so it should not be necessary to miss work or home commitments.

What actually happens when you have ultraviolet treatment?

Although the routine varies a bit with each individual case and with whether or not you take psoralen tablets, the physical process is much the same. The delivery units are like an upright sunbed with an array of tubes inside a private cabinet. You will need to strip off completely for the treatment, although men need to keep some minimal cover over their genitals. This could be a pair of minibriefs, a jockstrap or even a sock! You stay in the cabinet for only a matter of minutes and are then free to go. Most departments offering the treatment are very good at keeping to time so you arrive just before your time, have the treatment and leave without any undue waiting.

Why do I need to wear sunglasses on the days I have PUVA?

When the psoralen is taken by mouth, it is absorbed through the gut and affects more than just the skin. The eyes are also made more sensitive to light, which can cause cataracts to develop. To protect your eyes, you must wear glasses that filter out the ultraviolet rays as soon as you take the tablet. These need to be worn for the rest of the day. If you feel uncomfortable wearing sunglasses all day, you can get spectacles with clear glass that filters out ultraviolet light, but make absolutely certain that they are the right type. You should be able to get your glasses tested – to make sure they are filtering out the ultraviolet rays – in the dermatology department where you are having the UVA therapy.

More and more people are having the psoralen applied directly to the skin by lying in a bath of psoralen solution before the UVA treatment. Even then, enough of the drug may be absorbed to make the eyes sensitive and at risk so sunglasses are still needed.

Why do doctors offer treatments like PUVA with a slight risk involved when the end result isn't very good?

We would hope that the days in which doctors were accused of playing 'god' are gone. These days, the relationship between you and your doctor should be much more of a partnership as you have a right to know about all the available treatments and the risks involved so that you can play your part in deciding which one is best for you at any given time. We used to use the term 'compliance' to mean the way in which a patient stuck to the instructions for using a treatment; now, however, we use 'concordance' to indicate an agreement between the patient and the doctor about how and which treatment to use. You should be able to discuss with your doctor the benefits and possible risks associated with any treatment offered to you. Few options are risk-free, and the final decision about whether to go ahead should be yours.

PUVA and its risks are very well understood, and for most people it can work well, clearing the skin and delaying the return of their eczema. All patients having PUVA are carefully counselled about the risks, and most of them agree that these are acceptable. The bulk of the risk comes from the ultraviolet light, but in some circumstances the psoralen can cause problems. If there is a chance of damage to the liver from heavy drinking or because of a history of jaundice, the psoralen can cause extra damage. In such instances, blood tests are needed to make sure that the liver is working normally before using the treatment.

I have been offered narrow-band UVB treatment. What does this mean?

UVB contains quite a wide range of wavelengths (290–320 nanometres (nm)), and although it can be useful in eczema, it has never been as useful as PUVA. In the past few years, a more defined form of UVB (311 nm) has been developed – hence the name 'narrow band'. This seems to be almost as effective as PUVA without all the drawbacks of taking the psoralen, which makes it much easier to use. In addition, although PUVA may have a slightly higher rate of success, if your skin clears with narrow-band UVB, it will stay clear (in remission) as long as it would have done with PUVA. You have the treatment in the same way as with PUVA, by standing in a special cabinet containing UVB tubes – like fluorescent light tubes but made to emit only the UVB. Each treatment course involves a session every 2 or 3 days for 5–8 weeks.

Is narrow-band UVB treatment safer than PUVA?

Yes, it is. Because you are not using a psoralen, you will not have any of its possible side-effects, including the risk of developing cataracts if you do not wear the special glasses on treatment days. It can therefore be used in children and in pregnant women. Narrow-band UVB is still thought to increase the risk of skin cancer but not the dangerous melanoma type, whereas PUVA does increase the risk of melanoma and some other types of skin cancer. Because of this, you can have more UVB than PUVA sessions – 450 compared with between 150 and 200. Some people with very difficult eczema may need more than the maximum number of sessions of PUVA and they are advised to visit the dermatologist once every year just to have their skin checked for signs of cancer.

How do the doctors know how much ultraviolet light to give me?

This is a good question as we all vary in our reaction to ultraviolet light – as you can see on any beach in the summer! The dose of ultraviolet light used in narrow-band UVB and PUVA is worked out from the lowest amount that will turn your type of skin red (this redness being called erythema). This is known as the 'minimum erythema dose' (MED) for UVB, and the 'minimum phototoxic dose' (MPD) for PUVA as the added effect of the psoralen has to be accounted for. The redness lasts for 48–72 hours so treatment is usually given two or three times a week to allow the skin to recover between doses.

The starting dose is set at 70% of the MED or MPD and increased depending on the reaction to each treatment. If your skin does not show any redness, the next treatment will be 40% more than the previous one, but a little redness will reduce this increase to 20%. Once you start reacting to the treatment, it will be held at the same dose, but as you progress through a course, the dose is slowly increased to compensate for the tanning effect, which starts to block some of the ultraviolet light.

Is there any need to use my creams when having ultraviolet treatment?

It is well worth using a moisturiser regularly as the treatment may tend to make your skin dry, but most people like to have a rest from applying the active creams. If you are receiving UVB and it is not working as well as it might, the doctor might suggest using one of the active creams in between treatment sessions. There is also some evidence that applying a moisturiser before your UVB session helps the treatment to work better, but the moisturiser must be applied at least 2 hours beforehand to avoid any blocking effect on the skin. Some moisturisers contain a sunscreen and must not be used. It is certainly worth taking your moisturiser with you and applying some after each treatment session.

Treatment taken by mouth

This section covers evening primrose oil, systemic steroids, ciclosporin and azathioprine. 'Systemic' drugs are ones that may affect the whole body so they will have an effect on more than just the skin. Systemic drugs can be taken by mouth, by injection or by suppository.

With the exception of evening primrose oil, all these therapies are very strong and carry a number of potentially serious side-effects. Their use is restricted to severe eczema that has not responded well to other treatments, and they are usually prescribed and monitored only by doctors with expertise in their use. This does not just mean consultants as some GPs take a special interest in skin problems and can safely treat patients away from a hospital setting. Despite the need for monitoring to avoid side-effects, these drugs can make a dramatic difference to the life of someone with bad eczema.

Will taking evening primrose oil help my eczema?

There are several different types of evening primrose oil, made by various companies, and it is widely advertised for sale in magazines and newspaper colour supplements. Studies have been carried out to try to answer your question, but these have used a standard preparation that may be different from ones you see advertised, which is important in understanding the results. The active ingredient in evening primrose oil is gamma-linoleic acid, of which 40 mg is present in standard adult capsules and 80 mg in paediatric capsules (allowing children to take fewer doses). Many different makes of evening primrose oil are listed as having 500 mg of oil in them, but it is important to realise that this is the amount of oil and *not* the amount of the active ingredient. The results of the studies vary, some showing benefit and others none at all. The National Institute for Health and Clinical Excellence is a body that looks at evidence of how well various treatments work in an effort to prevent NHS money being wasted on treatments of dubious benefit. It classes evening primrose oil as having no proven benefit and no longer recommends it as a prescribable medicine in the NHS.

This advice is based on collecting together all the available studies so is true for large groups of people, but what is always difficult to refute is the benefit that some individuals may gain from evening primrose oil so we are happy to recommend that you give it a go, especially if your skin is very dry and flaky. Make sure that you buy the right preparation and try it for about 3 months maximum. You will need to take six capsules twice a day so it may work out expensive and you may end up being disappointed. Even if you seem to get better, you should stop taking the oil after 3 months as you might just have improved anyway and might stay better for a while. If your skin starts to dry and flake again very quickly, restart the evening primrose oil, and if your skin improves once more, this may well be a good treatment for you.

There are no concerns about side-effects as this is a very safe treatment. It is interesting to note that breast milk contains naturally higher levels of gamma-linoleic acid than are found in formula feeds for babies, but recent research suggests that breast-feeding may not be as good as was once thought for preventing the development of eczema in young children.

The dermatologist has suggested that ciclosporin may help my husband's eczema. Can you tell me more about this?

Ciclosporin is a drug used for severe eczema. It is a strong drug with potentially severe side-effects so you and your husband must make sure that you have a chance to discuss the risks and benefits fully with the consultant.

Ciclosporin acts by suppressing a chemical called interleukin-2 (IL-2), which is part of the body's immune system. Because ciclosporin does not affect all of the immune system in the way that steroids given by mouth do, the risk of infection while taking the treatment is lower. There does not seem to be any increase in the number of bacterial infections, but there may be a small risk of some viral infections such as herpes. It can certainly help severe eczema, some studies showing that over two-thirds of people taking it can expect an improvement, although maybe only a third do extremely well.

The two main serious side-effects that can occur are high blood pressure and kidney damage. Both of these seem to be reversible when the dose is decreased or the therapy is stopped as long as careful monitoring is carried out to pick up any problems as soon as they occur. This monitoring – with regular blood tests and blood pressure checks – is very important, and the treatment will be stopped if your husband does not keep being monitored. The problems with kidney damage seem to be more common in older people who have been taking the treatment for more than 6 months so some doctors now limit everyone's treatment to a course of up to 6 months, although a repeat course can be given after a break.

There are a number of lesser side-effects, including pins and needles in the fingers, mild tremor and nausea, which seem to improve despite continuing to take the therapy. Another problem is increased hair growth (which might be welcome for some people!) and an enlargement of the gums. The latter tends to occur in people with poor dental hygiene so regular dental check-ups are necessary.

My friend is taking ciclosporin after a kidney transplant. Why on earth is this used in eczema?

Ciclosporin is used in transplant medicine to help to prevent rejection of the transplanted organ. It acts by damping down the immune system in a rather more selective way than steroids do. Historically, somebody noticed that kidney transplant patients who also had the skin disease psoriasis found that their psoriasis got much better when they were started on ciclosporin. It became an approved therapy for psoriasis and was then tried for other inflammatory skin disorders such as eczema. The original studies looked at adults with eczema, but ciclosporin has also been studied in children, who seem to do well on it too.

My doctor says that taking ciclosporin can make it difficult to treat other conditions. Why is this?

Ciclosporin interacts with a number of oral treatments but not with topical ones. This interaction means that the side-effects of ciclosporin are more likely to occur or even that it may not work at all. This is because the other drugs can alter the levels of enzymes in the body that affect how quickly you get rid of ciclosporin – too quickly and it will not work; too slowly and you will get many more unwanted effects. You must tell any doctor who is treating you that you are taking ciclosporin as there is a long list of drugs it interacts with. Avoid buying over-the-counter drugs in shops where there is no pharmacist to advise you, and do not take herbal or other remedies whose effects are unknown. The common problem drugs are as follows:

- Antibiotics – erythromycin (a common antibiotic) should be avoided, but penicillin is safe.

- Antifungals – itraconazole is a drug used to treat fungal and yeast infections such as ringworm or thrush.

- Painkillers – aspirin and related drugs including ibuprofen (Advil, Brufen, Nurofen) and mefenamic acid (Ponstan) should be avoided, but paracetamol is safe.

- Antimalarials – chloroquine can interact, so avoid it if travelling abroad.

- Blood pressure tablets – diltiazem is one to avoid.

- Tablets for epilepsy – carbamazepine and phenytoin.

How long will I have to take ciclosporin for?

This depends on how severe your eczema is and how well you tolerate and respond to the drug. There are two ways to use ciclosporin – short-term/intermittent or long-term maintenance. In general, if your eczema is not too severe, you will be offered treatment for 4–12 weeks to try to clear your skin. Once it has cleared, the ciclosporin will be stopped, but you could have other short courses if it recurs. If your eczema is severe or keeps coming back very quickly after a short course, you will probably need maintenance treatment. In this case, you could start in the same way, but the dose will be reduced as your skin clears, down to the lowest dose that keeps it clear or keeps it at a level you are happy with.

My dermatologist has suggested a course of oral steroids to treat my eczema. How long should I take them for as I am worried about side-effects?

A short course of oral steroids is often used when eczema has got out of control as it can improve things quickly. Most dermatologists use them as a 2–4-week course, often starting at a high dose and then slowly decreasing the dose every few days. You are unlikely to notice any side-effects when steroids are used in this way. Indigestion or weight gain will occasionally occur, but this should settle down quickly as the steroids are reduced and stopped. Changes in mood – 'depression' or 'euphoria' – can also occur, especially if you have any pre-existing psychological problems, but again this should settle quickly as the steroids are withdrawn.

My child's asthma was so bad recently that the doctor treated him with steroid tablets. This led to a dramatic improvement in both his asthma and his eczema. Since stopping them, though, his eczema is getting bad again. Why can't he stay on this treatment?

Systemic steroids, rather than topical steroids, will usually produce a great improvement, or decrease, in eczema in both children and adults. There are a number of different ways of giving them, but you cannot avoid the side-effects if they are taken over a long period of time. For this reason, systemic steroids are usually given as a short course to try to control acute flares (more often in asthma than in eczema). Eczema will nearly always 'rebound' (worsen rapidly) if systemic steroids are withdrawn abruptly rather than tailing them off; courses for asthma are often given as a high dose for between a few days and a week without a reduction before stopping. Other treatments need to be put into place to prevent this rebound with eczema. These may include intensive emollients, other topical therapies, antibiotics and phototherapy. You could also ask your doctor whether any further courses that are needed for your son's asthma could be tailed off rather than stopped abruptly.

The side-effects of long-term systemic steroids that we worry about include:

- weight gain;

- bone-thinning;

- high blood pressure;

- diabetes;

- mood changes;

- thinning of the skin;

- growth suppression.

The last of these is a particular problem in children as severe eczema can also cause growth suppression. The most common steroid used as a tablet is called prednisolone; other steroid preparations, such as beclometasone and budesonide, are occasionally used. They seem to cause fewer problems in terms of weight gain and high blood pressure than prednisolone, but they can still suppress growth.

Another medication, called tetracosactrin (Synacthen), can be used, but this has to be given by injection. It is not a steroid but a hormone that makes the body's adrenal glands produce more of its own steroid; there are, however, side-effects similar to those of prednisolone even with this naturally produced steroid. It is usually only given as a one-off treatment boost in eczema that is difficult to get under control.

All long-term steroid therapy comes at a price – and we hope that your son's eczema is not severe enough to make this a price worth paying. It is particularly important to avoid this long-term therapy during puberty, when so much growth takes place. Our own view is that, for all ages, although short-term courses of systemic steroids are useful, long-term use should be the last line of therapy when all else has failed.

What is azathioprine?

Azathioprine is another very powerful medicine that suppresses the immune system. It works by damping down the bone marrow (which produces blood cells). It can also suppress parts of the bone

---

SAFETY FACTORS WITH ORAL STEROIDS

- All people taking oral steroids **must** carry a steroid card or bracelet giving details of the treatment; it is important for all medical personnel to have this information. Cards and bracelets are available from your pharmacist.

- People taking oral steroids should wait until they are off the treatment before being given 'live' vaccines such as MMR (measles, mumps and rubella), polio (the liquid given with the triple vaccine of diphtheria, tetanus and pertussis – whooping cough) and yellow fever (a travel vaccination).

- Oral steroids should not be stopped suddenly if they have been used for more than 4–6 weeks. Your doctor will give you a regime for stopping them gradually. Do not miss doses.

- If there is unrelated severe illness, surgery or trauma, the steroid doses may need to be doubled for a while – your doctor will advise you.

- Chickenpox can cause a widespread severe infection in children taking oral steroids. If your child has not had chickenpox and is on oral steroids, avoid contact with known cases of chickenpox or shingles. If such contact occurs, consult your doctor immediately for anti-chickenpox immunoglobulin therapy.

---

marrow that have nothing to do with the immune system so it can cause anaemia or blood-clotting problems. Azathioprine is used in many branches of medicine as an immunosuppressant for people with kidney transplants, arthritis, inflammatory bowel disease and various skin diseases. Its use in eczema has not been well studied, but most dermatologists are convinced, from long experience, that it works.

Azathioprine is used quite commonly in adults with severe eczema but rarely in children because of the greater concern over side-effects. As well as the worry about bone marrow suppression, there is a problem of liver damage so anyone taking it needs regular blood tests to watch for the first signs of this developing. Stopping the drug then will allow things to return to normal. Overall, azathioprine probably has fewer side-effects than oral steroids, and it is often used in combination with these if they are really needed as it allows a lower dose to be effective. Azathioprine is sometimes referred to as a 'steroid-sparing' agent.

My dermatologist offered me a blood test to see whether I could take azathioprine. Is it not suitable for everyone?

Part of the way in which azathioprine is broken down and removed from the body is through the action of an enzyme referred to as TMPT. Drugs have to be removed from the body so that they do not accumulate and reach toxic levels. About 1 in 300 people have low levels of TMPT, and this seems to put them at greater risk of bone marrow suppression. TMPT can therefore be used as a screening blood test before treatment, but this is not yet widely available. The benefit is a reduction in the number of monitoring tests you might have to have. At present, the recommended regime involves a full blood count every week for 8 weeks to check for bone marrow problems, with liver function tests at 2, 4 and 8 weeks and then every 2 months. If the TMPT test were found to be a safe predictor that a patient will have no bone marrow problems, these individuals would not need the full blood counts. The liver tests would still, however, be necessary as the way in which the liver can be affected differs from the effect on the bone marrow.

Are tablets used in eczema dangerous in overdose?

Yes – it is best to consider all tablets as dangerous in overdose, especially for children who might find a packet. Keep all tablets well out of reach of children, preferably in a locked cabinet.

6
Complementary therapies

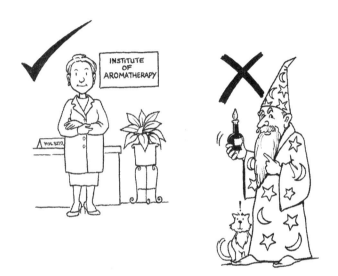

Introduction

Almost no modern medical book for patients or their carers would be complete without a section on complementary or 'non-conventional' treatments. It is, however, the most difficult area in which to give definite answers to questions. There is a wealth of information available on all sorts of different ways to treat eczema, and we are sure that there are many new treatments awaiting discovery or proper evaluation. It is this evaluation that makes this chapter very difficult to write.

Those who get better from complementary treatment are always very positive about it, as are the practitioners, and this can unfortunately raise the hopes of other people who will probably not get the same benefit. You will very rarely find people advertising the fact that a treatment has failed to work or made them worse. Most of the success stories are what we would call 'anecdotal evidence', and many anecdotes are needed to make a proven case. Proper scientific studies are needed to evaluate different therapies fully and prove their safety. It may not matter whether a patient chooses to spend money on a treatment that does not work, but it does matter if it makes them worse or ill in some other way. Every year, we hear reports of people dying from the toxic effects of herbal remedies, both Chinese and Western, so great care is needed in choosing a complementary practitioner.

Nevertheless, this approach to treatment is very popular, with around a third of adults who have persisting atopic eczema admitting to trying complementary medicine. One survey of children with atopic eczema attending a hospital in Leicester showed that 63% of them had tried or were intending to try it. This was not a very standard population as non-white ethnic groups were overrepresented and they had a great interest in Chinese and ayurvedic medicine to start with.

Choosing a safe practitioner

Most complementary practitioners work privately and are better than NHS doctors at 'selling' their treatment. They also tend to spend more time with patients, and there is undoubted benefit in being able to talk about your eczema and its impact on you. It can be very relaxing to talk, and we wish the NHS system could allow more time than it does for consultations. This is not to say that the only benefit from complementary medicine comes from spending money to buy 'protected time'. Some people do seem to get better, and as this includes children with eczema who might not gain as much psychological benefit from talking, a complementary option may be worth trying if a more conventional approach has not helped.

It is worth remembering that the term 'complementary' is used deliberately instead of 'alternative' as these treatments should sit alongside the standard first-line treatments and not replace them.

There are now professional bodies that regulate most forms of complementary treatment, and you should contact them before choosing a practitioner. They will have lists of people whose qualifications they feel are valid, but, unlike medicine, there is often no need to be registered with a professional body so you need to choose with care. Remember that you do not need any medical qualifications to work in complementary medicine so discuss your plans with your GP so that you can at least check whether the practitioner gets the diagnosis right.

How do I choose a safe complementary practitioner?

The Royal College of Nursing (see Appendix 1) has put together some very sensible guidelines for you to use when thinking about complementary medicine. This advice is also reflected in the guide produced by the Prince of Wales Foundation for Integrated Health (available on the Foundation's website; see Appendix 1), which also tells you much more about each type of therapy and which practitioners are regulated or about to become regulated.

You should always ask the practitioner:

- What are his or her qualifications, and how long was the training?
- Is he or she a member of a recognised, registered body with a code of practice?
- Can he or she give you the name, address and telephone number of this body so that you can check?
- Is the therapy available on the NHS?
- Can your GP delegate care to the practitioner?
- Does the practitioner keep your GP informed?
- Is this the most suitable complementary therapy for your eczema?
- Are the records confidential?
- What is the likely total cost of treatment?

- How many treatments will be needed?

- What insurance cover does the practitioner have if things go wrong?

Then ask yourself the following questions:

- Did the practitioner answer your questions clearly and to your satisfaction?

- Did he or she give you information to look through at your leisure?

- Did the practitioner conduct him- or herself in a professional manner?

- Were excessive claims made about the treatment?

You should avoid anyone who:

- claims to be able to cure eczema completely;

- advises you to stop your conventional treatment without consulting your GP;

- makes you feel uncomfortable – you need a good relationship if you are going to get full benefit from the treatment.

In short, you should demand the same standards from the practitioner as you would from a NHS doctor and subject the claims to the same critical scrutiny that is increasingly applied to NHS treatment.

Aromatherapy

I would like to try some aromatherapy. Friends have told me that the massage is very relaxing so I thought it might help me cope with my eczema. Would this be a good idea?

It really depends on how bad your skin is and how much 'normal' skin you have to be massaged. Aromatherapy involves the use of essential oils, which are aromatic (scented) and are extracted from the roots, flowers or leaves of plants. These oils can cause problems if massaged into the skin when you have eczema as you could be sensitive or even allergic to them. Massage is the usual way of using the oils and can be, in itself, very relaxing. If you do not have widespread eczema, it could be worth discussing it further with the aromatherapist. As with many new things you might want to put on your skin, we would recommend that any oil used is tested first before having the full massage. The simplest way for you to do this is to apply a little bit of it to somewhere free of eczema, such as your forearm, for a few days to rule out any chance of sensitivity.

Reflexology

What is reflexology, and can it help?

Reflexology is a massage therapy that uses acupuncture points on the feet that represent different parts of the body. The feet are massaged with talcum powder, and you do not need to take any other clothes off if you are self-conscious about your skin. As long as your feet are clear of eczema, it seems to be a safe treatment. You may have found that one problem with eczema is that other people may not like to touch your skin so the contact involved in reflexology can be very nice and reassuring. This in itself seems able to influence the disease as a positive attitude can help your body to fight it.

Chinese herbs

Chinese medicine is said to have made great advances towards helping various diseases by looking at them as a whole-body problem and using herbs to adjust the balance. I would like to try a Chinese herbal treatment but am not quite sure how to go about it – can you help?

Chinese herbal treatments come in two broad categories: creams, and preparations taken by mouth. The latter are most commonly used in eczema and have been subject to some trial work by traditional doctors. There seems to be some evidence that they can be beneficial in eczema, but studies have been quite small scale and need further evaluation. It is unlikely that this treatment will become available on the NHS in the foreseeable future as the licensing of drugs and similar items takes many years and is very expensive. This is necessary to try to exclude any products that might have dangerous long or short-term side-effects.

Several points need to be taken into account when considering Chinese herbal medicine:

- There is *no* good evidence that Chinese herbs cure eczema, but they may provide some benefits.

- Chinese herbs are not always safe as they can cause inflammation of, and damage to, internal organs such as the liver and kidneys in the short term. The long-term side-effects are unknown.

- The raw ingredients or herbs are not under any form of quality control so the chemical composition can vary enormously. Different countries of origin, times of year picked and storage conditions of the herbs can all have an effect on quality.

- There is a similar lack of control over the 'doctors' who sell the herbs. They are not medically qualified Western doctors under the control of the General Medical Council. Many are responsible, but you must remember that anyone can sell these herbs. A lot of money can be made if you think that the weekly cost can be £50–£60 per patient per week.

- Preparation of the herbs at home can take up to 2 hours as you have to boil them to make a liquid that you drink. It is recommended that you make a fresh preparation each time you take the treatment, which is often twice a day. The resulting black liquid has to be drunk but, unfortunately, usually tastes foul.

Recent reports ranging from undeclared potent steroids in Chinese herbal creams to deaths from kidney failure have highlighted the potential dangers of these preparations. There are calls for better regulation and more research, which are echoed by the reputable practitioners themselves. Chinese herbs undoubtedly seem to have helped some individuals so we hope that further research is possible to try to isolate an active ingredient or ingredients that could be used in a more controlled and safe way. In the next few years, we may be able to recommend a range of herbal treatments, but at present we would caution against them. If you do decide to go ahead, discuss this decision with your GP as it may be prudent to have some regular blood tests to make sure that your overall health is not suffering.

Other herbal treatment

Are there any non-Chinese herbal remedies?

Yes, there is a strong tradition of Western herbal medicine, with roots going back into folklore. There seems to be even less published work on this form of herbal treatment and very little scientific evidence that can be accepted by those with a conventional approach to treatment. Once again, however, most herbalists will spend time taking a careful history, and the creams that they use are often soothing with good moisturising properties.

Many of our modern medicines are of course derived from the study of traditional plant-based remedies, but an active ingredient has to be identified and thoroughly tested to ensure its safety before it can be licensed as a drug and be available on prescription. This may ignore the beneficial effects of a group of extracts working together so there will always be a place for this complementary approach.

You must remember, however, that your skin, and the skin of most people with eczema, can be very irritated by contacts with plants, and side-effects are possible. Check that any herbalist you visit is backed by a professional body, and test any new cream on a little bit of unaffected skin for a few days before you use it on your eczema. One herbal preparation that has been studied more than most – and has been compared with hydrocortisone in some trials – is camomile. There does seem to be some evidence that it has a specific action in improving eczema in addition to a simple moisturising effect; this is probably an anti-inflammatory action. Tea-tree oil is also growing in popularity and has useful antiseptic properties, but it has not been well studied in eczema.

Is it worth taking hemp seed oil?

There has been quite a bit of interest in hemp seed oil as it is high in polyunsaturated fatty acids such as omega-3, which are known to play a part in keeping the skin and nails healthy. One well-conducted study in which taking 30 ml of hemp seed oil a day was compared with taking 30 ml of olive oil was reported in a reputable journal (the *British Journal of Dermatology*) – olive oil was chosen as it looked much the same as the hemp seed oil so that patients would not know which product they were taking. The hemp seed oil gave rise to a significant improvement in atopic eczema, but it is not clear whether the oil would help any other types of eczema.

I am 24 and have had eczema since childhood. A local store recently suggested that I should try Wau Wa cream, which was described as a herbal cream from Ghana. Can you tell me anything about it?

Wau Wa cream claims to be made from petroleum jelly and the juice of the Wau Wa plant from Ghana. The most important thing to say about it is that a sample was analysed in 2001 and found to contain clobetasol – the same steroid that is in our most potent topical steroid. No wonder that there were people who used it and found that it worked! As with some other non-standard preparations, many different formulae may be used to make the 'same' product, but this is one of several 'herbal' remedies that have been found to contain steroids. We also know of cases of severe worsening of the eczema, which seems to arise from an allergic reaction to the plant extract.

Homeopathy

My friend sees a homeopathic doctor instead of an ordinary GP. What is homeopathy, and would it help my eczema?

Homeopaths believe that the symptoms of a disease are actually the body's way of fighting the illness. Rather than trying to reduce the symptoms with treatment, homeopathy tries to work with the body and add to its own healing powers. The 'remedy' prescribed is a minute dose of a substance that, in a normal dose, would produce the same symptoms in a healthy person. The remedy is produced by diluting the substance many times so that no more than a trace is present, and the resulting treatment is safe and usually free of side-effects, although there is a chance that your eczema might get worse in the initial stages of the treatment – this is referred to as 'aggravation'. It is very difficult to say whether your eczema would be helped by homeopathy. It might just be a case of giving it a go, but, be warned, it will involve a long-term approach to treating you – there are no quick fixes.

I visited a homeopathic doctor, and he seemed to spend more time asking questions about me than about my eczema. Why was this?

Homeopaths take a different approach to finding the 'right' remedy for you so often ask questions that seem to be much more about 'who you are' and 'what kind of person you are' than about your eczema. This approach can seem very attractive as it sets the eczema in the context of the type of person you are and exactly how you react to it. If the homeopath is going to give you a remedy that helps your body to heal itself, he feels he has to know what type of person you are. To try to understand this better, look at the following factors involved in how a homeopath would assess you as being suitable for treatment with a sulphur remedy as opposed to graphite or arsenic, which are other commonly used dilutions for eczema:

- the local pattern of eczema and how you react to it – extensor surfaces, extremely itchy or burning, feels good to scratch, scratch until it bleeds;

- things that make it worse – heat, especially when in bed;

- your mental make-up (the type of person you are) – assertive, argumentative, untidy, flamboyant or scruffy in dress;

- general comments about you – hot, rarely feel the cold, hot smelly feet, likes spicy food.

As you can see, you will be asked lots more about yourself before a remedy is chosen! One other recent example was a lady who hated to wear anything around her neck and was 'uncomfortable' with snakes. She was treated with Centrix contortrix, which the homeopath said 'came from an animal in the snake family'.

Is seeing a homeopath very expensive?

Homeopathy is one of the complementary treatments that you can have on the NHS: there are five homeopathic hospitals in Britain – Bristol, Glasgow, Liverpool, London and Tunbridge Wells. You and your GP need to decide between you whether you can be referred as your GP is governed by the policies of the local health organisations such as Primary Care Trusts and Local Health Boards. If this cannot be arranged, or you feel that it is too far to travel, you can see a practitioner privately; charges might start from around £30. As you do not need a prescription for homeopathic remedies, you could buy them directly from a pharmacy. Some pharmacists have qualifications in basic homeopathy and could advise you about what might be worth trying. You can get more information from the British Homeopathic Association (see Appendix 1).

What is ayurvedic medicine?

This is an ancient Hindu system of healing that is based on both 'naturopathy' and homeopathy. It also looks at 'body types' and has a concept of 'humours' that represent the five elements and their qualities. A consultation will involve procedures such as taking the pulse, observing your manner, skin and tongue colour and taking a description of your life and habits. A practitioner will then give you advice about diet, detoxification, plant and mineral treatments, the environment you live in and 'rejuvenation' therapies. This therefore gives you advice on how to live your life in the belief that you can be made to 'fit in' with the environment and laws of nature, leading to better health. There seems to be more of a danger that you will be encouraged to give up all your existing medication, but this will depend on the individual practitioner. The Medicines and Healthcare products Regulatory Agency has also recently warned about the inclusion of heavy metals in some ayurvedic medicines, meaning that they are not safe to use. More information can be obtained from the 'Safety of herbal medicines' page on the Agency's website.

Acupuncture

How is acupuncture supposed to work?

There is not really enough space here to fully answer such a big question. We are not experts in acupuncture but can give you the sort of explanation we might give to our patients. This is based on the theories of acupuncture, but although it might sound convincing, the results may not be as good. You can get more information from the British Medical Acupuncture Society (see Appendix 1).

Acupuncture uses points on the body that are stimulated by needles in the belief that this helps to clear excessive amounts of 'heat', 'damp' and 'wind' from the body. Practitioners see eczema as being characterised by redness and itching of the skin with crusting, scaling and blisters. They then diverge from conventional medicine by seeing these characteristics as being due to a mixture of problems with 'heat', 'damp' and 'wind':

- Heat is seen as causing the redness and inflammation.

- Damp reflects an overaccumulation of body fluids in the skin, leading to blisters.

- Wind is a little less straightforward but is seen as something that moves from place to place and can appear and disappear suddenly. Eczema with severe itching is seen as having a strong 'wind' component.

Although generalised chronic skin diseases are not thought to respond well to acupuncture, eczema with a definite allergic component can do, and it does seem to be able to reduce the sensation of itching.

Hypnotherapy

I successfully stopped smoking with hypnotherapy. My partner often says that I keep scratching my skin out of habit. Could this mean that my eczema has made me addicted to scratching and that I should try hypnotherapy?

This is a very good, logical question, and many readers will sympathise with you in feeling that they just cannot stop scratching. Many people feel that scratching can actually be a stimulus to keep your eczema going so anything that can reduce it is worth trying. There have been some studies of hypnotherapy and eczema that have shown benefit in decreasing the need to scratch, although little objective change was seen in the skin over the short period of the study. We do not think it unreasonable, however, to suggest that if you feel better about your skin and scratch it less, your eczema will improve slowly in the long term.

Some GPs have an interest in hypnosis, and it is relatively easy to learn a simple form of self-hypnosis. This can involve visualisation techniques in which you imagine that you 'see' a thermostat type of control that can be used to turn down the urge to itch as you would turn down the temperature using a real thermostat. If the idea of hypnotism does not appeal to you, you could look at the related techniques such as 'Neuro Linguistic Programming' as written about by, for example, Paul McKenna.

Conclusion

In summary, many people benefit from a complementary approach to treatment. Whether this is because of the extra time taken in consultations and the *whole-person approach* or because it is a really effective therapy is still open to debate. If your eczema gets better without any adverse effects, does it really matter? We feel, however, that it does matter because the only way in which these different approaches can become available to all is through acceptance into the NHS, and much more scientific evidence is needed for that. Whether the necessary research will take place is doubtful: it is a very expensive process, and money can only be made from a patentable new drug, not from a natural remedy.

7
Feelings, family and friends

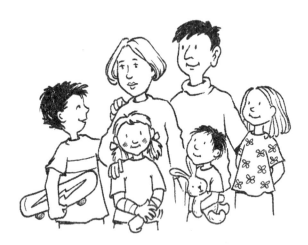

Introduction

It is impossible to consider the severity of eczema without taking
into account the effect it is having on an individual's psyche and
well-being. In this chapter, we talk about some of the emotional
and psychological aspects of having eczema and how this may
affect the individual, as well as the friends and family around them.
One recent study into the emotional effects of eczema is called,
rather appropriately, 'Isolate', which comes from its 'real' title –
the International Study of life with Atopic Eczema. Two thousand
people were interviewed across several European countries; 60%
of them had atopic eczema, and 40% cared for children with the
disease. We believe that the findings can also be applied to the other
forms of eczema unless they are very localised and easily treated:

- 33% said that eczema had affected their work/school, home and social life;
- 14% said that their career progression had been affected by eczema, whether through a limitation of choice of career or poor performance at interview;
- 36% found that flares affected their self-confidence;
- 51% felt unhappy or depressed during flares;
- 21% admitted to difficulties in forming relationships;
- 41% of those in established relationships said that they felt awkward about partners seeing or touching their bodies;
- 30% of patients and carers said that eczema had an impact on the lives of other members of the household;
- only 26% said that their doctor had discussed the emotional impact of eczema with them.

Emotional aspects

I am becoming very depressed and cannot concentrate on anything. I am losing sleep and feel I cannot take this any longer: it is affecting my work and personal life. Emotionally, I feel a wreck and need more help.

It sounds like you are going through a difficult time with your eczema. If your eczema is bad and you are losing sleep, it can certainly make you feel tired, irritable and more emotionally charged. Visit your doctor or nurse and review your treatment regime to see whether any modifications can be made to improve the control of your eczema. As you are not sleeping, it may be helpful to try a sedating antihistamine at night; try to take it regularly over a few nights to re-establish a better pattern of sleep.

Try also to talk to friends, family and colleagues at work: they may well be concerned and may have noticed that you are 'not yourself'. Support from those around you can be a real boost, and this may help you through this difficult time. It may be necessary to take some time off work; discuss this with your GP as he or she will be able to suggest other mechanisms of support or even a course of treatment for depression.

It may be helpful to join the National Eczema Society (see Appendix 1), which has fully trained information staff and both telephone and e-mail helplines. The Society will also be able to tell you whether there is a local support group in your area.

Does stress make my eczema worse?

Stress and other types of emotional arousal can certainly make eczema worse, and it is sometimes thought that children with eczema are prone to stress. Some common emotions that contribute to this are anger, sadness and feelings of guilt, all of which can be related to having itchy, red skin. The emotional stress tends to lead to increased sweating, which irritates the skin and triggers itching so the eczema gets worse. It is possible to get trapped into a vicious circle in which the worry of having eczema can lead to sweating and increased feelings of itch, which in turn cause increased worry and concern about what is happening. There is also some evidence that if you are not someone who copes well with stress, you may be more likely to suffer from hand eczema.

It depresses me to think that there is a link between my eczema and anxiety. Can you advise on any new approaches I could try?

It has been shown that there is a link between eczema and anxiety/stress. If you are able to identify your stressors and the situations that provoke your anxiety, you have made the first step in learning to cope with stressful events. Awareness will enable you to manage stressful situations more effectively.

It may also be useful to investigate relaxation techniques (such as special ways of breathing) and coping strategies, by remembering a stressful event and how you coped at that time, and then thinking about what you could have done differently. This will help you to approach new situations more confidently. Your GP should be able to refer you to a counsellor or psychologist if you need further help. You may get trapped into a vicious cycle of not coping, having negative thoughts, seeing your eczema worsen and then having even more feelings of not being able to cope. A psychological technique called cognitive behavioural therapy can be very useful in breaking this cycle by helping you to move away from the negative thoughts.

It is also worth talking to your specialist about having a 'back-up' plan, for when you know you are going to be stressed and your skin will flare, by having the necessary, stronger treatments available immediately; you may then feel a lot less anxious about the stress making your eczema worse.

Is there a connection between hyperactivity and eczema?

This is a difficult question to answer accurately as this has not been well studied. Psychological factors are certainly important in eczema. When stressed or upset, people with eczema scratch more and the eczema worsens, but the role of hyperactivity is less clear. In general, children with eczema are more likely to be introverted than extroverted. A point to consider is that the antihistamines used in eczema can occasionally cause stimulation and hyperactivity rather than the usual response of sedation. If this is the case, the antihistamine should be stopped or changed. There is certainly no evidence that eczema causes hyperactivity directly. One other possible mechanism is the disturbed sleep that many children with eczema get: a lack of deep, relaxing sleep has been linked to hyperactivity and other behavioural disorders in children.

Friends and relationships

My husband has very bad atopic eczema, which is making him angry and upset. I feel afraid and alone, and I can't even touch him to comfort him because it hurts so much. What can I do to help him?

This response is unfortunately a coping mechanism for some people and may be more of a problem with men, especially if they feel frustrated by previous ineffective treatments and do not express this very well. You need to talk to someone to overcome your feelings of being afraid and alone before you can start to help your husband. Contact the National Eczema Society (see Appendix 1), who can let you know if there is a local support group in your area. Your GP may also be able to put you in touch with counselling services.

Support groups can be extremely helpful by providing information and introducing you to people who are having similar experiences and will therefore understand what you are going through. This will help you to support your husband and encourage him to talk about how upset he is feeling. You could then move on to discussing whether he has accessed all the help and advice he needs from his GP, a specialist nurse or a consultant dermatologist. Taking a fresh look at current treatments and their effects can often improve a seemingly hopeless situation. If your husband would allow you to put on some of his creams, this could help in restoring some intimacy to your relationship.

I have never got over the psychological problems that eczema has caused. It affects my confidence and how I see myself; relationships are impossible as I fear rejection because of my eczema – should I try to speak to someone about this?

Yes it certainly sounds as though you would benefit from talking to someone. The National Eczema Society is a useful resource, and there are national support groups such as Changing Faces that deal with the psychological aspects of poor self-image. The addresses are in Appendix 1, and your GP may be able to help with information about any local groups. It is common for people with chronic eczema to feel this way. It may be necessary for you to explore your feelings with a counsellor who will be able to help you work through these issues in your own time or to explore more formal psychological therapies such as cognitive behavioural therapy.

You may find it useful talking to your GP about a specialist referral to achieve a better control of your eczema. This obviously would not resolve all your issues, but if your skin is more manageable and less inflamed, this will help to improve your self-esteem. It is often worth considering what you would realistically like to achieve and then make a list of the best outcomes for you before consulting a specialist so that you can discuss with the specialist how these outcomes can be achieved. It is very important for anyone treating you to know what your personal measure of success is going to be.

My confidence is low no matter how my friends and family are supporting me. What can I do about it?

You are not alone. Eczema is a chronic condition and as such can have an impact on how we see ourselves and deal with certain situations. When your skin flares, it is visible to others, and some patients feel frustrated when others draw attention to the eczema, feeling that they have to explain why their skin is red and angry.

It might be helpful to think whether there are certain situations that seem to affect your confidence more than others and try to list the aspects that trouble you the most. It can be very useful to talk to a specialist (such as a counsellor) about how you feel: friends and family can offer great support, but it is sometimes easier to talk openly about personal anxieties to someone you do not know.

My son is 17 years old. I am worried that he doesn't seem to have many friends and recently, when his eczema was very bad, he refused to leave the house. How can I help him?

The first step is to talk to your son and find out whether he feels that this is a problem. Some teenagers prefer to keep a small group of friends, or perhaps find making friends difficult regardless of any health problems. Do encourage your son to talk openly about his feelings and try to highlight specific problems. He may, for example, have had some difficult experiences at school, perhaps with teasing or bullying, which may cause him to be more reserved or cautious about new friends.

If your son finds it difficult to discuss this with you, encourage him to talk to another member of the family or his teacher or tutor, or seek support from a group such as the National Eczema Society (see Appendix 1), which has a leaflet for teenagers about dealing with eczema. Through discussion, you may be able to pinpoint why he feels concerned about leaving the house. Once you have done this, it is possible to work through concerns and anxieties so that he can move on from his present situation.

Eczema can cause misery for the sufferer as well as adding stress to other family members so do not be afraid to seek help and support from your GP or other members of the health-care team. Your GP will also be able to provide advice about other health professionals available for referral, such as clinical psychologists who are trained to help people with chronic conditions requiring extra support. It is possible to learn ways of thinking about and responding to various problems, such as chronic disease, that makes them easier to bear – these are called 'coping mechanisms'.

Family conflict

Since my daughter developed eczema, my whole life has revolved around her. Does this happen to other families? What can I do?

Indeed it does, and knowing that you are not alone is often a help. You could consider making contact with other families to share your feelings and worries. The National Eczema Society (see Appendix 1) can be a useful source of support.

Children can be very manipulative even without an illness to work with. Think of your response when your daughter is scratching. Will you stop doing everything else to deal with her? If you do, what message might this give to her and other members of your family? It is issues like these that may need the skills of a psychologist or family therapist. If you find you need help, start by talking to your GP on your own without your daughter.

You do not say how old your daughter is or who else is in the family. It is important gradually to hand over control of the management of eczema to children as they get older so that they can take more responsibility for their own problems. Start with emollients and perhaps leave the active treatments like topical steroids until you are sure that your daughter will use them safely. Other family members could also be involved in her care so that you stop feeling that the problem is all yours.

My husband is 27 years old and suffers badly with his eczema. One of our children has reached an age when he asks more questions about his dad's skin – this upsets my husband and he covers himself up. Is there anything I can do?

First, talk to your son, telling him what eczema is and how it affects the skin, and try to explain that dad does not feel comfortable talking about it at the moment. If your son feels more informed, he might be less likely to probe his dad with further questions.

Second, tell your husband the approach you have taken and explain to him, being sensitive and mindful of his needs, that your son also has needs, including that of reassurance as he is perhaps worried about his dad. Your husband should see it as a sign that his son loves him and wants to understand and help. If he could move to a point where he could allow your son to apply some of his emollients, this would be a great success.

Finally, eczema can have a great impact on how we see ourselves and how we feel others may see us. Support and encourage your husband to talk more to you all as a family about his eczema, but also be aware that he has developed ways of coping with his eczema and perhaps your son's questions are challenging your husband's tried-and-tested coping mechanisms.

My elderly mother lives with us and has developed terrible eczema over the past year. We are controlling it fairly well with the creams the doctor gave us, but the problem is that I feel exhausted. It is always me who helps to apply the creams – my husband and teenage daughter refuse to help. What can I do?

This is a difficult situation: you feel that you are taking the full burden of your mother's care yet your husband and daughter are reluctant to help. This may be due to a number of reasons:

- They may not feel confident about applying the treatments; they may view you as being very proficient and may worry that they will get it wrong.

- They may resent the time you need to spend with your mother rather than them.

- There may be other frustrations about the change in family dynamics since your mother moved in.

- Your husband may not feel able to have such intimate contact with your mother so may have to find other ways to help.

You need to talk to your husband and daughter and express how you feel; they may not be aware that you would like help or what is involved. You also need to talk to your mother and see how she would feel if your husband helped with treatments. An alternative might be to involve another female family member such as a sister. If this is not possible, many GP practices now have health visitors for the elderly. They should be able to offer practical advice and support, although they will not be able to apply the creams for you. You should also make sure that your GP knows how much strain you are feeling. It may well be possible to design a less intensive skin-care regime that will ease some of the burden.

Home life and routine

Our cat Fred has been with us for years. In the day he sneaks upstairs and sleeps on our bed – I am sure this makes my husband's eczema worse, but he doesn't agree. I am not suggesting we get rid of Fred, but should I keep him downstairs and off the bed?

Yes, we would agree that it is probably best for Fred to sleep downstairs and have limited access to some areas of the house.

Ban him from the bedrooms and where the eczema treatment is normally carried out. Generally speaking, pets with fur, hair or feathers are not a good idea with eczema, but we would rarely advise to get rid of an existing pet because of the psychological impact this would have. Careful thought is, however, needed when Fred dies and there is the temptation to replace him. The problem with cats is not with the fur itself but with a protein in the saliva, and you only have to watch the cat washing to realise that this is all over it.

Here is some general advice:

- Never allow pets on or under the bed.

- Do not allow pets near any bed linen.

- If you are sitting or kneeling on the floor, lay down a cotton sheet or throw to prevent contact with carpet fibres and animal hairs.

- If you need to handle the pet for grooming or stroking, it is best to wear cotton gloves.

My son is very attached to his teddy. Should I try to swap it for something less irritant to his eczema?

If your son is 'very attached' to his teddy, this will probably be very difficult. Soft toys can be a problem for children with eczema as they harbour house dust mite, but, as mentioned in Chapter 4, the exact role of the house dust mite in making eczema worse is not clear. Ideally, all stuffed toys should be avoided, but this can be very difficult indeed. If children do have soft toys, the following measures will be helpful in reducing any effect from the house dust mite:

- If possible, wash the teddy at a temperature higher than 55°C.

- Some toys cannot withstand this temperature so put them in a plastic bag and freeze them for 6 hours to kill any house dust mites. Then wash them according to the manufacturer's instructions.

- Try to get two or three of your son's favourite soft toys so that he always has one with him while the other is in the freezer or the wash.

- Hang the teddy outside on the line when it is sunny; the sun kills house dust mites.

This advice can be modified for household plush or fabric items and for personal clothing/accessories such as hats and scarves.

Having a toddler with eczema running around, I find it very difficult to know the best time to tackle the housework. Do you have any advice?

With young children, especially ones with eczema, developing a good routine is usually quite helpful considering the amount of time involved in cleaning and general housework. It is better to carry out vacuuming and dusting when your child has an afternoon nap or perhaps in the evening when you could get your partner to help.

Vacuuming disturbs the house dust mites in soft furnishings, which could be irritant to the child's skin. Damp-dusting is more beneficial than using polish, especially in your child's bedroom.

8
School

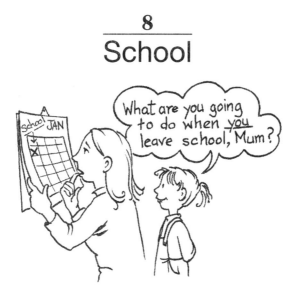

Introduction

School plays a major part in children's lives, but sadly for those with eczema, starting school can be the first time that they feel different and come up against teasing, bullying and prejudice. Many people still see eczema and other skin diseases as being 'infectious' or caused by a lack of hygiene. You may also find that you can have as many problems as your child because of adverse comments from parents.

Informing the school

Do I need to tell the school about my daughter's eczema?

No, you do not 'need' to, but you will probably find that your daughter has fewer problems if you can have a discussion about eczema with the teachers. They can then be on the look-out for problems such as teasing and bullying, and will be aware of the problems some activities at school may cause – and how to overcome them. You can also take the opportunity to ensure that the school understands eczema and correct any mistaken beliefs.

Should the school or my son keep the creams when he is at school?

Without knowing more details about your son, this is a difficult question to answer. Most of the active treatments for eczema (e.g. topical steroids, tablets) are used once or twice daily. The only exception to this is some antibiotics. This leaves your son's moisturiser and soap substitute as the only creams that that he will usually need at school. You should find out the school's policy and make sure it allows for easy access to creams for washing the hands. Most schools will keep prescription drugs that need to be given regularly, but they should have a more flexible policy towards creams – similar to asthma inhalers. You need to make sure that your son is happy and confident about using his creams and that he can have some privacy at school when he feels the need to apply them.

My son has a very bad habit of scratching when he is bored and left to his own devices. What will happen at school if the teacher doesn't notice him?

You need to discuss your concerns with your son's teacher. You may well find that he is usually so absorbed in activities at school that he does not have time, or forgets, to scratch. It would be worth suggesting that your son sits somewhere in the classroom away from a sunny window, radiator or other heat source so that he does not feel itchy from being too hot. Make sure that he has some moisturiser readily available to soothe his skin if he becomes itchy and that he has time to apply it. If there is an area that is persistently scratched, you could use some tubular stockinette bandage over emollients to protect the area. Do not fall into the trap of getting the teacher to stop him scratching by telling him off – negative feedback can do more harm than good.

Coping with irritation

My son's hands are constantly exposed to water, paints and sand in the nursery he attends. Is there anything I can do to minimise the damage caused by these?

Water play is a fun learning experience for children, but the water itself can have a drying effect on the skin. This may be alleviated by adding some of the bath oil your child usually uses to the water or by applying a thick, grease-based moisturiser to his hands prior to wet play. These measures will reduce the soreness and dryness of his hands, but it is important to reapply the moisturisers to the hands once wet play has finished, as well as regularly through the day. For play with sand, paint and glue, fine cotton gloves can be worn; these can be bought from a chemist or purchased through mail order (ask the National Eczema Society for advice; address in Appendix 1).

It will also be important to keep nursery staff informed, ensuring they are aware that soaps and detergents will irritate the skin and that a soap substitute should be used. Your son should have a good supply of soap substitute and moisturiser available at his nursery. Bear this in mind when requesting prescriptions from the GP: either ask for double quantities so that one tub can stay at nursery, or ask for some smaller tubes of moisturiser to keep at different venues. Alternatively, you can use some small tubs and decant the moisturiser out.

My daughter loves reading and writing, but the eczema on her hands is sometimes so bad that she can't hold a pen.

Learning to write will be difficult with sore, cracked, dry fingers. Carrying out more intensive skin treatments during this phase will improve the skin. This can be particularly helpful overnight so that the skin is less dry and more flexible in the morning. Use plenty of greasy moisturiser at night. Cotton gloves or stockinette mittens can be applied to hold the moisturiser in place, helping it to work more effectively, and prevent scratching through the night. If there are cracks and splits on the fingers, paste bandages can be helpful to occlude these areas overnight. It will also be vital to continue moisturising the hands during the day, perhaps using a cream base, which will be less greasy and allow your daughter to hold a pen.

In difficult cases, cotton gloves with the fingertips cut off can be used for school. This will protect the hands while leaving the fingertips exposed to grip a pen but might make your daughter feel more different. Alternatively, discuss with her teacher the possibility of waiting a couple of days before resuming writing activities or seeing whether a computer would be an acceptable alternative as she could still practise her spelling and sentence formation.

I find it very difficult to deal with my 5-year-old son's eczema now that he has started full-time school. Lots of his school play activities include things that seem to make his eczema worse or at least difficult to manage.

Starting full-time school can be an exciting time but can cause some difficulties for children with eczema. It is important to build up good communication with the staff at school: it may be helpful to make a special appointment with your child's teacher to discuss his eczema and any concerns that you might have. The National Eczema Society (see Appendix 1) produces School Activity Packs (foundation to year 3, years 4–7 and years 8–11) as well as a Teacher's Guide, and it is well worth giving the school a copy of the relevant ones. It can be helpful to provide the school with a written skin-care regime for your son and link this to clearly labelled pots of emollient to use during the day. You could also highlight on this list some common problems, such as the need to apply moisturiser frequently after certain activities or what to do if your son is hot and itchy.

It might be useful for the teacher to talk to the other children in the class about eczema and make them aware that eczema is not contagious. It would also be very helpful to let teachers and other parents know that your son should avoid skin-to-skin contact with anyone with a cold sore as this might lead to eczema herpeticum.

The teacher complains that my daughter falls asleep during lessons. Is her eczema to blame?

Sleeping during the day could be related to a number of reasons. First, if your child's eczema is flared, dry and itchy, she may find herself awake during the night scratching. Persistent disrupted sleep can take its toll, and your daughter may be flagging during the busy school day. Second, sedating antihistamines, which are an anti-itch medication, are often used at night in conjunction with a topical treatment regime. If your daughter is taking these, it may be useful to review the dosage. It may be too high and need adjustment, or the timing may need to be changed as giving the drug too late in the evening can leave your child drowsy the next day. If you feel that none of these factors applies to your daughter, it may be worth considering whether anything else, such as bad dreams, is disturbing her sleep.

Swimming and other sport

My daughter started swimming with school at the start of this term. I have noticed that, after swimming, her skin is drier and she complains of itching and soreness at night. I don't want to exclude her from swimming but I am worried that it's making her eczema worse.

Swimming can certainly have a drying effect on eczematous skin, leading to increased irritation; your daughter does not necessarily have to avoid swimming. In fact, it is important, in order to avoid feelings of exclusion and being different, that your child participates in all the activities that one would expect in a normal school life.

The main problem with swimming is the chlorine, which has an extreme drying effect on the skin. Showering afterwards can be helpful, although this is sometimes a hit-and-miss affair at school. It is important that the teacher is aware of your daughter's need to moisturise her skin well after swimming and the fact that she might need some privacy to do this. In addition, you can compensate for the drying effect by giving your child an oily emollient bath when she returns home, applying plenty of moisturiser afterwards: the thicker greasy moisturisers are the best. These can also be applied to the skin prior to swimming, thus providing a protective barrier for the skin. Unfortunately, this will make your child's skin slippery so she must take care to avoid slipping in the pool and supervisors need to be aware that if she needs assistance out of the pool, she will be slippery to handle.

There may be times when swimming is best avoided in the short term, for example when the eczema is in a flared state, weepy or infected, as the skin is then more prone to irritation. This will also avoid the possibility of your child feeling embarrassed at getting undressed in front of others.

My son won't take part in PE at school because of his eczema. What can we do?

First, sit down with your son and find out why he dislikes PE – some children just don't like it. Alternatively, this could be related to his eczema, such as concerns about his skin's appearance and what other children will say, or the fact that participating in PE makes his skin more sore and uncomfortable. Children can sometimes be cruel, picking on others who are different by teasing, name-calling or even bullying. If you suspect this, it is vital to discuss it with your son's teacher, who will be able to talk to the other children involved. Most schools have a policy to deal with bullying. It might be that your son will be happier if he can wear a long-sleeved cotton T-shirt and tracksuit bottoms rather than the traditional shorts and T-shirt.

If physical activity is aggravating the eczema, suggest that he has a cool-down shower and applies plenty of moisturiser afterwards.

My son enjoys football club at school, but the eczema on his legs becomes very inflamed after playing. I don't want to stop him playing, but what can I do to avoid this?

During sports, the skin becomes hot owing to body motion and perhaps also friction from fabrics against the skin. To reduce irritation to the skin, ensure that it is well moisturised – send a small quantity of his usual moisturiser in his sports bag so he can apply some before and after playing.

Sweating can also irritate the skin so encourage your son to wear clothing that keeps him cool and comfortable. Shorts are generally cooler, but he may prefer tracksuit bottoms if he is conscious about how his eczema looks. Chat to him about this and find the best compromise. It might be worth experimenting with different fabrics. Cotton is usually better than synthetic fibres as it is cool and will tend to absorb moisture, but some people find that cotton sportswear chafes. Furthermore, if your son wears shin pads, check the inside layer that goes next to the skin in case it is tending to rub or irritate. It can be helpful to use a layer of tubular stockinette (Tubifast or Comfifast) between the skin and the shin pad. It is now possible to get stockinette garments; the tights (which are footless) are very helpful for sports such as this or for other hobbies, for example horse-riding, gymnastics and dancing.

Finally, it might be useful to encourage your son to take an oily emollient bath when he gets home and top up with plenty of moisturisers.

Statement of Special Educational Needs

I have recently visited the school that my son is due to start this year to explain about his eczema, which is severe. They have suggested that I apply to have him 'statemented'. What does this mean, and how do I go about it?

The term 'statemented' refers to recognising your son's needs and highlighting any extra help that he may require. The 1991 Education Act stated that all children should, wherever possible, be integrated into mainstream schools. Statements were therefore developed that highlighted 'special educational needs'.

We would advise the parents of any child with special needs to find out as much as possible about statements from their Local Education Authority and use the statement to get the best for their child. Your son's age is irrelevant as you do not have to wait until he is of school age before starting the statement process. The Department for Education and Employment publishes a booklet called *Special Educational Needs – A Guide for Parents and Carers* (see Appendix 2), which outlines the procedures and explains the jargon used. Most people think of special educational needs as relating only to children with learning difficulties, but this applies equally to children with severe physical problems, and eczema can unfortunately fall into this category. The National Eczema Society (see Appendix 1) can provide a letter explaining about eczema and the effect it can have, which can accompany your application.

Exams

My son has to sit his exams this summer. He has not missed any school, but I am worried that his eczema may interfere with these exams. Is there anything I can do to help him?

The first thing to say is that research studies have shown that most children with eczema perform as well at school as those without eczema. There is, however, the possibility that the stress of the exams and the hot summer weather may act as triggers to cause a flare of your son's eczema. Ensure that he has a cool shady room to revise in and will have a place in the examination hall away from sunlight. Chat to your son about how he feels, and suggest what treatments he could use if his skin does start to flare. Review his treatment regime and intensify the topical therapy to get the best possible control of his eczema. Ask if he is happy with his moisturiser or whether it is too greasy. Lighter creams are better in the summer months. Try to avoid systemic treatments such as oral steroids or antihistamines that may interfere with sleep patterns or concentration.

If he does have a bad flare that you and he feel has prevented him from producing his best work in an exam, discuss this with his tutor. You may be able to get the examining board to take this into consideration. They will usually require a confirmatory letter from his doctor even if you can alter his treatment yourself to cope with it. A doctor cannot write a letter saying that your son's eczema has been a problem if he or she did not see him at the time so try to be proactive and discuss this with your GP before the exam period.

For children with moderate-to-severe eczema, it is possible to apply to the appropriate examination board(s) for dispensations that may include:

- extra time for pupils who have difficulty writing because of eczema on their hands;

- permission for the pupil to record his or her answers on tape;

- relocation to a special needs department;

- relocation to a hospital ward.

9

Social life and holidays

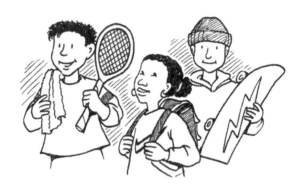

Introduction

This chapter is very important. It may be that it overlaps with some of the answers given in other chapters, but it allows us to include problems specifically relating to social life, such as make-up, hairstyle and general grooming. As people with eczema know, it is often the impact that eczema can have on quality of life that makes it so much of a problem. We hope that some of the answers here will help people to live life as fully and 'normally' as possible despite their skin problems. As with some of the other advice given in the book, it probably applies much more to people with atopic or contact eczema than some of the other types. It is important to realise that even eczema that is confined to the hands can have a profound effect on quality of life – up to 70% of adults with hand eczema report that it hampers their leisure activities.

Sporting activities

Why do I feel so itchy after playing football?

Any sport or activity that leads to sweating can cause itching. Indoor sports, such as karate, five-a-side football, squash and badminton tend to be worse than outdoor sports because the sweat does not evaporate as quickly as it does outside. Sweat itself is very irritant. Think of the stinging that sweat can cause if it drips into your eyes. Sweat has exactly the same irritant, stinging effect on the sensitive skin of eczema.

Having said that, you need to carry on with your football and try to lead a normal life. If you do become itchy after football, try a lukewarm shower to help you cool down, using a soap-free emollient wash. Some of these come in the same types of container that are used for shower gel so it need not be obvious that you are not using an 'ordinary' shower gel. Dry off gently without rubbing your skin too much, and apply a light moisturiser as soon as you can. If you have a choice about what kit to wear, choose a cotton shirt or one of the new fabrics that draws off sweat – you can get T-shirts made of this material that you can wear under your sports shirt.

I am heavily involved in sports and find that my eczema gets very irritated on the crease of my forearms when I get home after I have been sweating. I find that showering afterwards does not seem to help very much. What else can I do?

This sounds a troublesome problem. The flexures – especially in front of the elbow – are a common site for eczema so this is probably why you only have a problem there. It is undoubtedly linked to your sweating so you need to try to lessen the irritant effect that the sweat can have. You could try a sweatband worn over or just above the elbow to see whether this soaks up enough sweat to help, and combine this with using a very light moisturiser applied to the crease before you start exercising. One of the lotions, for example Dermol lotion, would be ideal. This should not increase the amount of sweating in the way a greasier one might do, and should act as a barrier. You should still take a lukewarm shower using a non-soap cleanser as soon after exercise as possible.

Can I go swimming even though I get eczema?

Yes, you can if it is a form of exercise you enjoy. Chlorinated water can be irritant to the skin so it is probably best to stay out of the water when you have a flare. You can minimise any irritation by following a simple routine:

- Apply a moisturiser before going into the pool.
- Shower as soon as possible after coming out of the water and try to put up with lukewarm water.
- Reapply some moisturiser.

We have heard tales of people being asked, quite unreasonably, by pool attendants not to swim with eczema because they feel it is 'catching'. If you are faced with this situation, the National Eczema Society (see Appendix 1) will be able to provide you with a letter explaining that eczema is not catching.

Make-up and hairstyle

My daughter wanted to have her face painted at a local fête. She has eczema, but it has never been on her face. Is this OK?

Yes, this will probably be OK. There are some people who are allergic to something in face paints, but this is quite rare, especially in children. You could see this time what type of paint they use and try it out on her forearm or somewhere without any eczema for a few days to see whether there is any reaction, and then allow her to have her face painted next time. This may, however, be totally unrealistic, so as long as her face is clear, let her behave like all her friends and have her face painted!

Is it OK to use make-up when you have eczema?

Yes, this is all part of making your life as normal as possible. If you have eczema caused by contact problems, discoid eczema or eczema related to varicose veins, there will be no problem at all. If you have atopic eczema from childhood there might be some problems but they are usually easily overcome. Try any new make-up on the inside of your forearm for 2–3 days; if there is no reaction, it should be fine on your face. It is worth seeking out one of the 'hypoallergenic' make-ups, such as those by ROC and Clinique, as they are less likely to contain chemicals that you might become allergic to with prolonged use. If your eczema flares for any other reason, you will need to be very careful as anything can irritate when your skin is inflamed.

Is there any problem with having my head shaved? Will it cause eczema?

No, it is unlikely to have any effect on your eczema even if your scalp is affected. If it is, you may actually want to think twice about it as it may make your eczema more obvious to other people. Hair can be very good at covering up scalp problems. If your scalp is free from eczema, go for it as it is all part of normal life.

I have had eczema since I was a baby. I would really like to get my ears pierced. Will this be safe?

Yes, it should be, as long as you don't have active eczema in your ears at the time of the piercing. Some people worry about developing nickel allergy from earrings, but this in fact is no more common in people with atopic eczema, which is probably the type of eczema you have, than in those without. You should insist that you are provided with studs that do not contain any nickel, for example good-quality gold, British sterling silver and platinum. Most of the problems with earrings are probably caused by irritant eczema from the build-up of soap and shampoo around them when showering or bathing. It can be very difficult to thoroughly rinse around earrings so it may be better to remove them before hair-washing, showering or bathing.

I have African/Caribbean hair and want to straighten it. Will this cause problems with my eczema?

Hair-straightening is popular with African/Caribbean people, as is the use of hair oils and treatments. There is no reason why you should not try to straighten your hair, but you may have to take a few precautions. Three different techniques are used: heat, acid and alkali – the latter two are known as 'chemical relaxers' and have a longer-lasting effect. They all act by breaking down the disulphide chemical bonds that make hair naturally curly and only affect the hair that is there at the time of treatment, not new hair as it grows.

Heat. Combing with hot oils was popular but has recently gone rather out of fashion because it has to be repeated more frequently. A new range of hair-straightening tongs with ceramic or glass plates that are heated electrically are very easy to use but also have only a temporary effect over a day or two. They are designed for home use, and you could use them even if your eczema is active on your scalp as no oils are involved.

Acid. This uses an acid chemical called ammonium thioglycolate that is also used to create the opposite effect in a perm.

Alkali. The chemical used here is sodium hydroxide.

Both chemical methods also involve the use of neutralising chemicals to stop the reaction. If the chemicals are left on too long, they will cause a chemical burn on the scalp whether or not you have any eczema there, so it is important to use an experienced hairdresser to ensure that the chemicals are used correctly. The straightening can last for weeks. All the chemicals are potentially irritant so should not be used if you have active eczema on your scalp, but they are OK if you have eczema elsewhere but your scalp is clear.

Is it safe to wear artificial nails?

Sculptured artificial nails are growing in popularity, with a great increase in the number of nail bars seen on the high street. These nails are made of acrylics and can cause problems with the development of allergy. If you do react, you might notice eczema developing on your fingertips and perhaps on your neck and eyelids, which are areas that many people touch frequently, and often subconsciously, with their nails. In extreme cases where the problem has not been recognised, there can be long-term damage to the natural nail itself. The acrylics can also cause hand eczema in the technicians working in the nail bars. This is not, however, a very common problem, although the incidence seems to be increasing. Hospital departments doing patch-testing for eczema might see only a few people with this each year. You will have to decide whether you want to take a small risk given that if you start to develop eczema and stop using the nails immediately, you will not have done any long-term damage.

Computers

I spend a lot of time at a computer for work. Could this make my eczema worse?

No, there is no evidence that computers, or any other bits of electrical equipment, can trigger or cause eczema to flare. If you are using the keyboard with both hands, you will not be scratching so this may even be good for your skin! You may already have realised that you need to be careful with your choice of moisturiser when using the computer – something too greasy will make your fingers slip on the keys so stick to a light lotion or cream that may need to be applied more often.

Visiting friends

My 4-year-old daughter has recently been invited to a friend's birthday party. She is on a dairy-free diet for her eczema. How can I be sure that she won't be given any dairy products?

It is difficult to be completely sure about this, but you should speak to the friend's parents to see whether they are prepared to help. Remember, though, that having completely separate food may make your daughter feel different or singled out. Don't be too worried, however, because an occasional break from her diet is unlikely to cause any problems.

Talking generally without knowing the precise details of your daughter's eczema, exclusion diets tend to be more beneficial in children younger than she is. At this age, we would probably be encouraging you gradually to reintroduce dairy products as her hypersensitivity may well have reduced as she has grown older. Many people seem able to eat a full range of foods even if they initially had a problem with one or two. Any reintroduction of food must be done slowly and in small amounts over a few months so this could be an opportunity to start the process off. Try discussing it with your daughter as well – she may be able to help you to decide and be willing to take the risk that her eczema might temporarily flare if she is still hypersensitive.

It is worth just stressing here that severe allergies that cause swelling of the lips, wheezing and fainting are a different matter. Perhaps the most well known of these is the reaction to peanuts, but it can also happen with eggs or fish and these foods **MUST** be **completely avoided** at all times if they have been identified as the cause of this different and much more serious reaction.

Holidays

Is there a mosquito repellent suitable for people with eczema?

Never forget that the 'physical' methods that prevent mosquitoes from getting to your skin are the best things to use first. These include appropriate clothing – long-sleeved cotton shirts, long trousers and socks (especially in the evening) – and a mosquito net at night. These should be used in addition to any repellent.

Mosquito coils and burners can also be useful at night if a net is not available, but perhaps the best and safest 'non-contact' device is a plug-in repellent that works off an electrical socket. All of the mosquito repellents put directly on to the skin, especially the liquid ones, which are alcohol based and sting, can cause some irritation if your eczema is active. If you are keen to use these repellents, try the usual test before your holiday of applying a little bit to a test area on your forearm for a few days. Another approach is to use ankle and wrist bands that are impregnated with a repellent called DEET – they do not seem to cause too many problems.

We want to go on a family holiday but are worried about different things in the environment and in hotels that might cause problems. We all have, or have had, eczema, but it is mainly a concern for the children.

Holidays should be a time for everyone to be relaxed so we understand why you are concerned. Most people, including children, seem to find that their eczema improves on holiday – probably owing to a combination of sunshine, relaxation and a change of environment. You will have to be a little careful in choosing the environment, based on your own knowledge of what tends to cause problems for your family. It is worth taking a few general precautions such as checking ahead with accommodation and avoiding old, traditional hotels that might have deep-pile carpets and heavy curtains to harbour house dust mites. Similarly, you should try to avoid feather pillows and duvets – some people find it useful to take their own pillow cases and a cotton sleeping-bag liner, especially if they are concerned about scratching in the night and leaving spots of blood on the sheets.

Extremes of air-conditioning and central heating can be a problem, but most hotels seem to allow you to alter the room temperature. You cannot, however, alter the outside temperature, and hot, humid conditions can be very uncomfortable for someone with eczema as sweating and using lots of cream do not go well together. Cold, windy conditions will tend to dry out your skin more quickly, but it is easier to cope with this by using more emollients.

Overall, seaside holidays seem to be best for children with eczema even though sand can be irritant if not washed off. It is important to try to avoid always choosing a holiday on the basis of a child with eczema as this can cause tension in the family if other people would prefer more variety.

Finally, remember to take enough treatment on holiday with you – extra moisturiser is often needed and can be difficult and expensive to obtain overseas. If you are flying, pack some of your treatments in your hand luggage in case you are delayed or your suitcases get lost! You might need to use more of a lighter moisturiser on holiday as this can be more comfortable in hot weather.

We are about to go on holiday to Spain. My husband still has bad eczema, and we realise we should use a sun-block cream in strong sunshine. Can you recommend any suitable ones?

He may find that his eczema improves on a sunny holiday as long as the weather is not too hot and humid. Ultraviolet rays are recognised as being able to damp down inflammation in the skin, which is why they are used as a treatment for some people (see Chapter 5). You are, however, quite right to be concerned about strong sunshine as too much is bad for the skin, causing more rapid ageing and increasing the risk of skin cancer later in life. If your husband has skin that never tans but just burns, he will need to cover up and avoid the sun most of the time. Seeking out shade and wearing long-sleeved cotton shirts, sun hats and sun blocks should be encouraged. If he does tan, some cautious sun exposure can be safe and beneficial – he could start with a short time each day and build it up to get a tan and avoid burning. Everyone should avoid the middle of the day – do like the Spanish and have a long lunch indoors followed by a siesta! Be particularly careful that you do not sit in the shade only for ultraviolet rays to be reflected off white buildings or water.

A large number of sun-block creams are available nowadays to protect you when out in the sun, but remember that they are the last line of defence and should not be used as a way of staying out longer. The protection is not complete, and you should not believe anything that claims to be a total sun block – even a completely opaque cream will rub off and stop working. Look for a product with a sun protection factor (SPF) of at least 15. This means that you would get the same exposure to ultraviolet B (UVB) rays in 15 minutes using the cream that you would get in 1 minute without it. There is actually very little difference in protection above 15 as creams need to be applied regularly, especially after swimming or sweating, which tends to dilute them and lead to their being rubbed off. Any product should cover UVA as well as UVB rays. This is indicated by a star rating system, four stars indicating the best protection. UVA penetrates more deeply into the skin, causing long-term damage, but does not cause burning. Therefore, blocking just the UVB to prevent burning might mean that you will stay out in the sun longer, which is dangerous as you will get more UVA exposure.

Sun blocks come in two types: chemical absorbers and physical reflectors. Reflectors are less likely to cause an allergic problem but can be less cosmetically acceptable as they tend to be more opaque in appearance. We do not have any strong views on which will be better for your husband so he may have to try a few out before you go away. Some creams are said to be waterproof, but 'water-resistant' may be a better term, as swimming will decrease their effectiveness, and they should always be reapplied afterwards.

A final point to remember is that sunshine is drying to the skin so make sure your husband packs extra moisturiser, with perhaps a greasier one than normal to use at night; he may, however, prefer a lighter one in the heat of the day.

Our son wants to go on scout camp. He has had bad eczema for some years, and we are worried about his treatments. Should we stop him from going?

If your son is old enough to go on scout camp, he should be old enough to apply his own treatments and may already be doing so. All children with eczema should be encouraged to start applying their own creams as soon as they seem able to as this encourages independence and a feeling of being 'in control'. In view of this, we think that it is really important for your son to go on the camp. The camp organisers will want to know all about his eczema as part of their own preparation, as well as to satisfy health and safety and risk assessment regulations. Talk it through with them and, if necessary, let them have some of the National Eczema Society's advice sheets (see Appendix 1 for contact details). Eczema is very common so you may find they have dealt with many similar children before. If you are still concerned, you could ask them to give you a ring during the camp to reassure you – without letting your son know that you are checking up on him!

Are there any special holidays available for children with bad eczema?

Yes, there is a programme called Peak, run by Asthma UK, that is supported by the National Eczema Society as it caters for children with asthma and related conditions – one of which is eczema (see Appendix 1 for contact details). Holidays are arranged during the school holidays all over the UK and in Jersey. A variety of age groups are catered for, and the aim is to provide a happy, safe environment for children to experience a variety of activities and sports and build up their self-confidence. The adult helpers tend to be a mixture of parents, medical personnel and staff from the patient organisations. Similar holidays are run in the USA if your child is a bit more adventurous.

Since we have booked our package holiday, we have heard from a friend that her child had problems joining in with the activities organised for children by the holidays reps. Will this be a problem?

It all depends on the severity of your child's eczema, the reaction of the individual holiday rep and the activities involved. The rep may be subject to a company policy or may be allowed to make his or her own judgements. Try to find out more about the company's approach before you go, and seek out the rep at the start to make sure that he or she understands that eczema is not catching, etc.

Is eczema something that needs to be declared on a travel insurance form?

Without knowing the details of the application form, it is difficult to say anything other than 'probably'. It is usually a chronic condition, so there is a chance that it might flare when you are away. As it is a 'pre-existing' condition, the company might try to wriggle out of paying for treatment abroad if you have not declared it. It is unlikely to lead to any rise in the premium.

Can we get access to medical care abroad?

This depends on which country you visit, but your travel agent or holiday company should be able to give you the correct advice. Medical attention is supposed to be free in all EU countries as long as you have certificate E111, which is available from post offices. Some of the newer member states may not, however, make it as easy as it should be to access treatment. From 1 January 2006, the European Union will use European Health Insurance Cards, and the E111 will become invalid. The Department of Health produces a useful booklet called *The Traveller's Guide to Health* (see Appendix 2).

10

Eczema through the ages

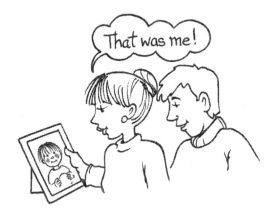

Introduction

As we grow older, our skin changes, and eczema sufferers will find that their eczema also changes over the years. This chapter aims to outline some of the common problems experienced at different times of life – a 6-month-old baby with atopic eczema may have very different needs and problems from those of a teenager who is experiencing an eczema flare or an elderly lady who has developed eczema on her lower leg.

Parents tend to ask whether their child will grow out of eczema, and many children will. The susceptibility to eczema is, however, part and parcel of our genetic system and will always be present; consequently, eczema can clear and present no specific problems over a period of years but can then return as a flare or as an irritant eczema, especially on the hands.

As our skin ages it becomes drier, and if we have this susceptibility to eczema, we can find that the skin becomes more irritable and sometimes inflamed. We often see eczema presenting in the elderly for this very reason.

Immunisation

Are there any immunisations my baby should avoid?

No, all immunisations should be given to children with eczema. As with other children, your doctor may delay the immunisations if your baby is suffering from an acute illness or has a raised temperature. A flare of eczema without general illness is not a reason for delay. Some children are still offered a BCG to protect against tuberculosis. Although this is no longer routine, it is given when there is a high risk of exposure to tuberculosis. This applies mostly to people in inner-city areas, children whose families have come from high-risk countries such as India and Pakistan, and contacts of cases of tuberculosis. The only precaution to take when given a BCG is to use normal skin rather than skin with eczema for the injection site.

My child has both eczema and asthma so he uses steroid creams and steroid inhalers. Is it dangerous for him to have immunisations?

No, the only reason for delaying immunisation because of steroid treatment is if the steroids are being given by mouth as tablets or medicine. In this case, the child will usually be too ill to have immunisations, but even when a course of steroids has finished, you should wait 3 months before the injections.

Children and adults with asthma should have an injection against influenza each year. This vaccine is prepared in eggs so should not be given to anyone who is allergic to them. If you feel that eggs have made your symptoms of eczema or asthma worse, you can have a skin-prick test to check this (see Chapter 2). Even if your son is allergic to eggs, it may be possible for him to have an injection under the supervision of a community paediatrician after referral from your GP.

School-age children

My daughter is smaller than other girls in her class. Could this be due to her eczema?

There may be a number of explanations for this. Small stature tends to run in families, and this is the most common reason why children are smaller than their friends. Eczema can cause growth suppression but only if it is severe and difficult to control over a long period of time. Other factors to consider with your daughter are whether she has been on a restricted diet and the medication she has been using. Steroids taken by mouth for longer than a few weeks can suppress growth. Topical steroids are normally without this side-effect unless a very strong steroid (group 2 creams; see Table 3 in Chapter 4) is used for a number of months. Growth delayed by eczema normally catches up when the eczema is controlled.

Make sure you seek advice from your doctor or health visitor as there are charts available to monitor your child's weight and height. If the professionals believe your daughter's values are outside the normal range and none of the above situations apply, your GP may decide to refer her to a paediatrician. Rare conditions such as food malabsorption and hormone deficiency may sometimes have to be considered.

Will my child grow out of her eczema?

There is a good chance that your child's eczema will improve or disappear altogether with time. It is difficult to predict accurately when this will happen, but about 50% of children with early-onset eczema (eczema starting before the age of 1 year) will have improved significantly by the age of 5, and more than 90% will have improved by the age of 18. If, however, the onset of eczema is later in childhood, especially if it appears in the teenage years, the outlook is not as good.

Teenagers

My teenage son gets eczema on his face and has recently started to shave. Which is the best shaving method?

Shaving can be a difficult issue, and the best method is often a very individual choice as some patients with eczema will feel that the electric shaver is the best, whereas others prefer a wet shave and may well report that alternative methods of shaving cause irritation and soreness. The actual shaving action itself can be quite irritant owing to the physical trauma on the skin.

If your son chooses to wet-shave, it is worth mentioning that the shaving foam, gel or cream can sometimes cause an irritant reaction on the skin. For wet-shaving, he should try the following. First, apply a thick layer of moisturiser to the beard area and allow it to soak in (this can take a few minutes). Then wet the face thoroughly and apply a generous amount of moisturiser or soap substitute as a shaving gel. Shaving gel or foam can be used, but this will tend to have more of a drying effect on the skin; it is worth having a go with the moisturiser or soap substitute if possible. Your son will find that these do tend to clog up the razor a little bit more quickly, but they can easily be rinsed away with warm water. Shave in the direction of hair growth, i.e. the direction in which the skin feels smooth, which will generally be downwards on the face but may be in different directions, especially on the neck. Next, rinse and dry the skin and apply more moisturiser. For wet-shaving, it is important to use a good-quality razor, for example one that is guarded by a wire mesh to prevent cuts. It is also important to change the blade regularly.

Shaving in the direction of the hair growth will leave the hair a little longer than shaving against the growth, but a closer shave will tend to leave more damage to the skin and potential irritation. It can also cause problems in those of African/Caribbean origin and others with curly hair as the curled hair tends to grow back into the skin, causing inflamed lumps that can get infected. If your son would like to try a closer shave, he could shave against the growth after shaving with the growth and then add a further application of foam, gel or moisturiser.

For dry-shaving, your son should get a good-quality electric razor. It is worth applying moisturiser before and after, but a longer time is needed before shaving so that the moisturiser is thoroughly absorbed and does not clog up the razor.

After-shaves should be avoided where possible or kept to a minimum as these are based on alcohol and can tend to cause stinging or drying of the skin.

My daughter is 14 years old and usually manages her eczema very well independently. This Christmas, however, we have seen a change. She became very upset as she received a number of gifts such as bubble bath, body lotion and perfume, which, because of her eczema, she feels that she is unable to use. She has become angry about her eczema, and I need to remind her to use her creams more often as she seems to skip treatment. I am not sure what to do.

This is a very difficult situation for both you and your daughter. I would suggest that, if possible, you sit down and talk to her about how she is feeling about her eczema and its treatment. I would suggest that your daughter feels frustrated by the need to constantly treat her eczema with an unrelenting regime of emollients; she may well be seeing her friends experimenting with different cosmetics, perfumes and toiletries, and she may feel excluded from this by her condition.

Talking through her feelings will help to pinpoint areas that are upsetting her. Perhaps you can together work through some mechanisms or techniques for her to manage her eczema effectively but still participate fully with her peers. She could, for example, try putting perfume on her clothes rather than directly on her skin and using her soap substitute rather than a cleanser to remove make-up.

If your daughter feels that she would like to experiment more with her toiletries rather than using just the prescribed brands, it may be helpful to try makes such as Clinique, Body Shop or Boots own-brand range, which offer hypoallergenic or sensitive skin products that are usually suitable for people with eczema. This will to some extent depend on how flared her eczema is at the time. If she finds a brand that particularly suits her, she could suggest to people who want to buy her presents that they could choose something specifically from that range.

One tip for her is to try out any new make-up or perfume for a few days on an area of her skin that is free from eczema – people often choose the inside of the forearm. If it does not cause any problem there, she could try it on other areas, avoiding any active eczema.

My teenager is fed up with using steroids to treat her eczema. What are the alternatives?

If your daughter is fed up with using steroids, she may be using them inappropriately. They are designed only for short-term use so she may not be using enough preventive treatment such as soap substitutes and moisturiser, or her eczema may need a stronger treatment. Anyone can get fed up with regular treatment, and teenagers do tend to rebel against any routines that are imposed on them or affect their developing individuality.

Without knowing the details of your daughter's eczema, it is difficult to discuss alternatives that might be relevant to her. If she just objects to steroids, she could try an alternative such as the topical immune immunomodulatory drug Protopic. Some herbal preparations, for example camomile, can help and are discussed further in Chapter 6. Other approaches include taking tablets or going to hospital, and you should read the sections on these treatments earlier in the book.

My 15-year-old daughter has for years had eczema affecting her elbows and knees. This has improved as she has got older, but recently she has developed bad eczema around her eyes. Why is this?

If her eczema is beginning to improve, it is unusual for it suddenly to appear at a previously unaffected site. It may well be that she has developed a genuine allergic eczema (contact eczema or contact dermatitis) around her eyes on top of the atopic eczema. The most likely culprit is eye make-up or nail varnish – as people frequently touch their skin around their eyes with their fingers. We would advise that your GP refer her to be patch-tested by your local dermatologist (see more about patch tests in Chapter 2).

My teenage son still has eczema and has begun to develop acne. Does he need to change his eczema treatment?

This is a tricky problem for him, and he is unlucky as it is somewhat unusual for acne and eczema to occur together. The type of eczema that causes most problems on the face is seborrhoeic eczema, but atopic eczema also occurs here. It is difficult to imagine how the skin can both be dry with eczema and greasy with acne, but the two conditions can happen on different parts of the face. Your son's eczema treatment for his face should be no more than a moisturiser and the occasional use of a mild topical steroid. A light moisturiser is advisable as it prevents clogging up of the pores.

If he uses topical treatment for his acne, he could have problems because many of the preparations contain alcohol or other substances that dry the skin. Your doctor can discuss how to use tablet treatment to manage the acne without making the eczema worse.

Work and careers

My daughter has set her heart on being a nurse, but she had eczema as a child. Is this likely to stop her from getting a job?

No, your daughter can still get a job as a nurse, but the following must be considered and discussed sympathetically with her. As a nurse, she will undoubtedly be at increased risk of developing eczema again, especially on her hands. This is particularly true if she had troublesome hand eczema as a child. Even if the eczema has been gone for many years, nursing inevitably entails frequent washing of the hands, which can cause irritation of the skin and make the eczema more likely to recur. If the eczema does come back during her nursing career, it may significantly interfere with the job, although using gloves to protect the skin, using an aqueous cream as a soap substitute for washing and regularly using a hand-moisturising cream may help.

These measures may not, however, be sufficient to stop your daughter developing bad eczema, and we are sorry to say that we have seen some nurses who have had to give up their chosen profession because of troublesome eczema. This seems a terrible waste of many years of dedication in training so we would advise you to have a long chat with your daughter, explaining the risks, and even arrange for her to talk things through with the nurse. You may mention that there are many worthwhile jobs in health care, such as physiotherapy, occupational health, management, etc., that carry a much lower risk of provoking a recurrence of her eczema.

My child has just seen a careers advisor at school. She has had bad eczema since she was a baby so are there any careers that she should avoid?

There are a number of careers that can make eczema worse or cause a recurrence of eczema in people who have grown out of it. The jobs that involve manual work and contact with irritants are the least desirable. The following might cause problems:

- hairdressing;
- catering;
- food-handling;
- nursing;
- floristry and gardening;
- engineering and garage mechanics;
- animal-handling;
- vet/veterinary nursing;

- building or working with cement;

- the armed forces as the medical entrance requirement may be difficult to meet.

We feel that it is important to sit down with your daughter at an early stage, explain the situation and see how she feels. It can be helpful to take the view that horizons have changed rather than necessarily narrowed, and it is better to deal with this problem at an early stage rather than after she has committed to a chosen career and has started the training. In general, non-manual jobs such as administration, computer-based work, journalism, film-making, singing, fashion design, teaching or any office-based work are most suitable.

If your daughter seems uninterested, try to arrange for friends in appropriate jobs to show her around their workplaces and take the opportunity of any work experience schemes available through her school. Other people she could talk to about her career include a doctor or skin specialist, university careers advisory services and the Disablement Employment Advisor, who can be contacted through your local JobCentre.

My son is about to leave school and still has eczema. Will he have to tell his future employers about his skin?

Yes, he is legally obliged to tell his employers about any medical condition, including eczema. Employers or their occupational health department may ask for other details to try to assess how severe the condition has been. In general, it is unlikely that having eczema will decrease your son's chance of obtaining most jobs, with the exception of those mentioned in the previous answer.

My eczema seems to have been troublesome recently. It becomes worse at work, and I am worried about seeing the occupational health people as they might stop me doing my job.

It can be difficult when you can recognise that work is a trigger for making your eczema worse, particularly if you have a fear that seeking help might cause you to lose your job. It is important, though, to remember that the occupational health personnel are there to maintain your health and safety within the workplace, and if there is some aspect of your work that is making your eczema worse, they can help you to investigate this in a supportive manner. In addition, they can give you more specific advice in relation to the type of job that you do; for example, if you are carrying out manual work, they will be able to ensure that you have the correct protective equipment, such as gloves.

If you feel that it is too difficult to approach the occupational health department, it may be helpful to make an appointment to discuss your eczema management further with your GP or nurse so that you may optimise your treatment and find a treatment regime that will deal more effectively with the types of flare that you are experiencing at work.

As mentioned in the previous question, certain types of occupation can tend to aggravate eczema more than others. If your job is in one of these at-risk categories, it is probably worth thinking about your practices at work and considering whether there are any ways of avoiding potential irritants. If your work is more administrative, the problem might be the physical environment in which you are working; many eczema sufferers, for example, find that air-conditioned offices can have a very drying effect on their skin. Humidifiers can occasionally be fitted in the office, but a simple solution is just to place some bowls of water around the area in which you are working – as the water evaporates, it will slightly increase the humidity of the environment. It is also important to ensure that you have a supply of your usual creams at work so that you can apply them when required.

Finally, if this problem persists, it may be worth asking your GP whether you could see a specialist with a view to going for contact patch-testing to see whether you have any contact allergies. This does not necessarily mean that you will need to change your job if the tests are positive: it will simply mean that you will know exactly what is causing your skin to flare so you can take measures to avoid this and your employers are obliged to help you.

I am a junior doctor and can manage my current hand eczema with emollients. However, I am due to carry on to a surgical placement. Can you offer practical advice on hand-washing, scrubbing-up and the use of alcohol hand rub?

It sounds as though you already have an effective treatment regime but, as you say, the surgical placement might well challenge this. General hand-washing with soaps can create a general dryness and irritation of the skin owing to their alkaline base, but surgical scrubs usually use much harsher agents. Surgical scrubbing will certainly exacerbate your hand eczema, as will the use of alcohol rubs.

Recognising the potential difficulty of the placement is the first important step. We would advise that you discuss this with your tutor as well as the occupational health department. Soap substitutes can generally be used for hand-washing. You may find that Dermol 500 lotion is useful. This comes in a pump-action container and contains antiseptic agents; it has been shown to be effective against MRSA (methicillin-resistant *Staphylococcus aureus*), a bacterium sometimes found in hospitals. It is important to clarify whether the occupational health department will be happy for you to use this to scrub up and as an alternative to the alcohol rubs.

In addition, it will be helpful to have a flare regime planned as frequent hand-washing can irritate anyone's skin regardless of eczema. It might be helpful to compensate with a greasy emollient and cotton gloves at night and a stronger steroid ointment to tackle flares as they arise.

I have developed facial eczema, which is made worse by occupational stress. I am 52 years old, and my doctor thought it was due to hormone imbalance, but my blood hormone level is normal and eczema was confirmed. Why has this appeared almost literally overnight?

Eczema can sometimes develop out of the blue. If it does, it is important to think back to your childhood: did you have eczema as a baby; have you always had dry or sensitive skin? This is often a precursor of eczema flares. Stress can certainly be a trigger that can aggravate eczema, and it sounds as if you are already aware of the stress. If it is purely related to work, it may be worth discussing this further with your employer or occupational health department. Alternatively, you could talk to your GP, who may be able to advise you about relaxation techniques and other ways of dealing with stress.

Furthermore, if you find that your eczema flares at work, it may be worth considering whether any factors in the work environment are causing either an irritant reaction or a contact sensitivity reaction on the skin. This depends on the type of work you do. Discuss it further with your GP, who will if necessary refer you to a specialist for advice and possibly patch-testing.

Relationships

My daughter is 15 and most of her friends have boyfriends. I am sure she would have a boyfriend but for her eczema. She won't talk about it to my husband or me. What can we do to help her?

This is a difficult problem, but there are probably a number of factors involved. We do not know how bad your daughter's eczema is, but even if it is mild, it is likely to affect her at this age. It is difficult enough at the best of times for children to deal with a changing body and emotions, and any minor blemishes such as warts or spots can assume great importance. Eczema on visible areas such as her hands or face could be devastating to her self-confidence.

Teenagers are frequently reluctant to talk to their parents. They often feel unloved and unwanted, and may blame their eczema for being the sole cause of their problems. Your daughter may become disillusioned and fed up with treatment and may now be using it less often. She may find some of the ointments too greasy and cosmetically unacceptable. The teenage years can unfortunately be very trying times for both teenagers and parents alike!

There is no easy approach to this problem, but if your daughter has a close family friend or relative in whom she confides, it may be worth enlisting their support. Your doctor, nurse or specialist may also be able to provide a sympathetic ear for her. A review of your daughter's treatment would be worthwhile anyway to try to find a treatment regime that suits her and that she is prepared to use. Finally, the National Eczema Society (see Appendix 1) may be able to put her in touch locally with other teenagers of the same age who have similar problems. She may be able to express herself more easily with them than with you. These measures may help to build up her self-confidence, but although you can facilitate this, she must be allowed to find her own feet at her own pace.

Hormonal changes – sex, periods, pregnancy and the menopause

My daughter has recently started having periods and finds that her eczema gets worse before each monthly bleed. What can she do about this?

Hormones can have an effect on eczema, and this can be an extra problem on top of all the other changes related to puberty. We are afraid that this area is poorly understood. It will be worthwhile reviewing your daughter's treatment regime with her doctor or nurse to optimise the control of her eczema and to devise an action plan for potential flares.

If the premenstrual flare is very severe, 'hormonal manipulation' might help, but this is still a controversial treatment and the way it works is not yet clear. Treatment might include the contraceptive pill, but this carries some risks, and you need to consider these carefully through a discussion with your doctor.

I am troubled with chronic eczema. Should this affect which method of contraception I choose?

Generally speaking, it is unlikely that you will have problems with any form of contraception. You should, however, be aware of the potential of latex allergy – this will result in problems using the cap or condoms. It is also possible to react to some of the spermicidal gels used with a cap.

Would it be dangerous to become pregnant while on eczema medication?

If the treatment is just topical creams, the answer is no – even though steroid preparations tend to carry a warning about pregnancy. The systemic therapies, prednisolone, ciclosporin, azathioprine and PUVA therapy **MUST** be avoided during pregnancy. All tablets should be avoided in the first 3 months of pregnancy if possible. If antibiotics have to be given, penicillin and erythromycin are suitable. Antihistamines can usually be avoided in pregnancy but are thought to be safe. Chlorphenamine (Piriton) is often used and is regarded as one of the safest.

If eczema herpeticum develops, oral aciclovir is recommended because it seems to be relatively safe and any risk is far less serious than leaving the condition untreated.

Since I became pregnant, my eczema seems to have become worse, and my worry is that I will pass it on to my baby when he is born.

We must first reassure you that having a bad eczema flare in pregnancy will not increase the likelihood of your child having eczema. Eczema is an atopic disease and linked with a family history of eczema, asthma and hay fever. If there is a history of this in your family, it is possible that your child's genetic make-up may make him or her susceptible to developing eczema – the stronger the family history, the greater the chance of this happening.

My hand eczema is particularly bad at the moment; it is extremely painful. The problem is that I am 7 weeks' pregnant and not able to use any steroid creams. What can I do?

Your eczema has probably become worse because you have stopped your steroid creams. It is generally felt that it is safe to use topical steroid preparations in pregnancy (see the question above). We recognise your concern about using medication in pregnancy, but without the steroid, the eczema is likely to persist.

To get the best effect from topical steroids, visit your doctor or nurse to discuss your emollient regime and see whether any aspects of this should be modified. You should also check that you are using the right amount of topical steroid on the affected area.

It is also worth considering general hand care, avoiding irritants and protecting the hands where possible. It is worth refining this now as, once you have a new baby, frequent nappy changes and hand-washing can often aggravate existing hand eczema.

I have had eczema since I was 25 years old, but over the past 6 months, I have developed eczema on my areola. I have Eumovate cream from the GP, but this doesn't make much difference. Could this be related to the fact that I have recently started on HRT?

It is difficult to say whether this is related to your HRT (hormone replacement therapy). Eczema can certainly be affected by changes in hormonal balance, as described in earlier questions, but there is no evidence to link exacerbations of eczema with HRT. We would suggest that you ask your GP to review this again. One approach would be to alter the treatment regime, increasing the greasiness of the moisturiser and changing the steroid cream to ointment. Next, consider whether anything is causing irritation in that area, for example friction from clothing or perfumed body spray. Finally, if the problem persists, it is important for your GP to confirm that this is eczema and, if there is doubt, refer you to a specialist.

The elderly

My mother, who is 81 years old, developed eczema 8 months ago. Why should she be troubled with a skin problem now when her skin has been problem-free for most of her life?

As the skin ages, it becomes drier. This dryness can lead to irritation, scratching and inflammation; as the barrier function of the skin is further altered by this, the skin continues to dry out even more. In some cases, the elderly can develop asteatotic eczema, which gives a dry, crispy, crazy paving pattern on the skin. This usually responds very well to an emollient regime.

My mother has bad varicose eczema, and when it flares, she insists in bathing her feet in cold water as this is the only relief. Is there any thing wrong with doing this?

Itch can be so unbearable at times that we come across all sorts of technique being used to reduce it. Your mother's approach will be reducing the itch – because of the cold temperature – but she may find that the itch restarts when her feet come out of the water. Soaking in plain water can have a drying effect on the skin, which may in the long run exacerbate the eczema. Alternatives could be to keep a moisturising cream in the fridge so that the cold cream can be applied when the itch is bad. A cream will be more cooling than an ointment as the water in the cream evaporates off the warm skin. A further option would be for your mother to try wet-wraps on her legs (as described in Chapter 4); she would need to discuss this further with her doctor or nurse and be shown the technique.

11
Practical concerns

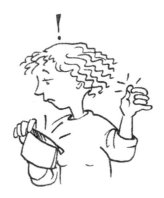

Introduction

This chapter covers some of the practical aspects of living with eczema. We will discuss some of the day-to-day issues, financial considerations and sources of further help and advice.

Financial considerations

I have very bad eczema. Am I entitled to claim any benefits?

Yes, you are, but we would advise you to seek help with filling in the forms involved so that you can bring out the full impact that the eczema has on your life. For any benefit claim or financial worries, we recommend that you seek assistance from your local Disability Benefits Centre (dealt with by the Disability and Carers Service, part of the Department of Work and Pensions; see Appendix 1); alternatively, a social worker accessed through your GP or hospital can advise you. The Citizens Advice Bureau (see Appendix 1 or your local phone book) can also sometimes provide information.

The *Disability Living Allowance* (DLA) is the first state benefit you should think about. It is not means-tested so your level of income will not affect the claim, and the allowance will not affect any other benefits that you or your family are claiming.

My neighbour cares for her father, who has terrible eczema. She said that they were able to claim for Carer's Allowance and Disability Living Allowance. Is this correct?

Yes, it could be. Carer's Allowance is a benefit paid to the informal carers of people who are severely disabled. You do not have to be related to, or live with, the person to claim this. You can claim Carer's Allowance if you are aged 16 or over and spend at least 35 hours a week caring for the same relative, friend or neighbour. He or she should be receiving, for example, Attendance Allowance or Disability Living Allowance (at the middle or highest rate for personal care). You cannot claim Carer's Allowance if you are in full-time education with 21 hours or more a week of supervised study or earn more than £82 a week after certain deductions have been made.

At the time of writing, the weekly rate is £45.70. This is reduced by the amount of certain other benefits, including the State Pension, that you might receive. You can find out more from www.direct.gov.uk.

I haven't been able to get specific benefits and find it difficult to cope with the expense of special bedding and extra laundry. Is there any other way of getting help?

You may be able to get a loan or grant from the Social Fund if you are currently receiving social security benefits. Contact your local Benefits Centre (see Appendix 1) to find out more details.

If it is your child who has eczema, grants are available through the Family Fund (see Appendix 1), financed by the government for families with severely disabled children. If, however, your child is not eligible for the Disability Living Allowance, it is unlikely that he or she would qualify for this.

My son will soon be 16. As he is on four different preparations on prescription, I am concerned about cost – will he continue to get free prescriptions?

If he is going on in full-time education to the age of 18 he will; if not, he won't if you live in England, Scotland or Northern Ireland. Wales is the exception because the National Assembly there has used its powers to keep prescriptions free until the age of 25. The costs of prescriptions can be a real concern for people with eczema because, unlike patients with epilepsy or diabetes, they are not entitled to free prescriptions.

If you need to pay for prescriptions, the most efficient way is to purchase a prepayment certificate. This is like a 'season ticket' for either 3 months or a whole year and will save you money if you need more than six prescriptions a quarter or 15 items per year. Your pharmacist, doctor or nurse should be able to give you a leaflet explaining how the scheme works. It is possible to order the certificate by post, telephone or Internet – these options allow the use of a credit card for purchase. It is also worth remembering that the certificate can be back-dated for a few days so it is worth getting a receipt for the initial prescription and claiming the cost back when the certificate arrives.

Washing clothes

The various creams and ointments have left grease marks on my clothes. Is there any advice on washing clothes?

Greasy ointments are particularly difficult to remove completely, even during hot-wash cycles. It is often best to use cream-based moisturisers during the day where possible as they cause less damage to clothing; greasy preparations can be used at bedtime when it is possible to use old nightclothes. If greasy ointments are used during the day, stockinette coverings can reduce damage to clothing. Biological washing powders are better than non-biological ones at removing grease and, provided the clothes are well rinsed, should not cause a problem with eczema.

I have heard that grease can damage washing machines. Is this true?

Yes, greasy moisturisers may cause the rubber seals on the washing machines to age more quickly. These seals vary in quality, both between manufacturers and within model ranges. If you are thinking of buying a new washing machine, it is probably best to write to the manufacturers and ask for advice as some seals are more resistant than others to this ageing.

We contacted Hotpoint, who gave us the following advice. Once a month, carry out a 95°C wash with no clothes in the machine, using biological washing powder because this helps to break down the grease and unclog the system. If this is not your usual choice of powder, do a second wash with your usual brand before washing your clothes.

I have repeatedly changed washing detergents. Are there any brands that you could advise me to use?

There is no one brand to recommend: any non-biological washing powder is acceptable. There is no need to go to a great deal of expense. An efficient rinse and spin programme on your washing machine is, however, essential. Research has shown that the soap residue left on clothes from insufficient rinsing, hand-washing or too much in one load of washing can be irritant to eczematous skin. An extra rinse cycle on the washing machine can be helpful. Fabric conditioners tend to be perfumed so should be avoided.

My doctor gave me a prescription for hydrocortisone 0.5% and said I didn't need a prescription as it would only cost a few pence. The chemist said that stronger versions were available off prescription but this mild dose was not so I had to pay the full prescription cost. Is this correct?

Yes, it all depends on if the drug is on the General Sales List (GSL), Pharmacy Only (P) or Prescription-only Medicine (PoM). GSL and P medicines can be sold over the counter at the discretion of the pharmacist, whereas a PoM cannot be sold in such a way. This can be very frustrating and expensive with items such as this. One option is to buy a prepayment certificate as described above. A further suggestion is to mention to your doctor or nurse that you pay for prescriptions and ask whether there is an alternative that you can buy over the counter. It is also worth remembering that, although some medicines are cheaper over the counter, many are not, and you may find it cheaper with a prescription, particularly for bath oils and emollients, etc. You could ask your doctor to prescribe enough to last 3 months as a way of reducing the expense of monthly prescription charges.

Miscellaneous

I saw on a website that a water softener might help. Would you advise buying one?

It is difficult to give advice on buying a water softener. Some patients with eczema find that it helps to improve their skin-care maintenance, but there is no specific evidence to support this. Water softeners can be expensive so if you are interested it might be worth asking the company whether you can have a trial period first to see if one is helpful.

I have contact eczema and have an allergy to latex and the chemical that rubber and leather are treated with. Finding shoes to which I am not allergic is a complete nightmare. Where can I find information about footwear that is not treated in the standard way?

First, ask for further information from your dermatology department, where you have probably had patch-testing to confirm your contact eczema. They should be able to advise you of what constituents you are allergic to. Once armed with this information, it may be best to contact a number of shoe manufacturers directly to ask whether their shoes meet your specification. We can see how difficult this must be for you, but once you find a manufacturer that can meet your needs, things will be easier. Contact the National Eczema Society (see Appendix 1), who can give you details of organisations that may be able to help you find suitable footwear.

I have recently been patch-tested and found I have a contact allergy to nickel. Do you know where I could get a kit to test my jewellery, keys, etc.?

Most good pharmacists should be able to advise you how to obtain a kit. They are not available on prescription, but hospital departments are occasionally able to supply them if a company has given them some sample kits.

Research

Are there going to be any breakthroughs in eczema treatment in the near future?

It seems unlikely that there are going to be any major breakthroughs in the near future, but there may well be some changes in the way we use existing treatments and in the different combinations tried at the same time. There will undoubtedly be advances in emollient therapy with the addition of different antimicrobial agents to help combat infection. The search is on for an 'ideal' emollient that could be applied only once a day but stay effective for 24 hours.

New immunomodulatory agents will be developed, building on the experience gained from pimecrolimus (Elidel) and tacrolimus (Protopic). Changes should reduce the initial irritation and try to boost the potency. Pimecrolimus may be produced as a tablet to give it more effectiveness.

A greater use of systemic agents is being encouraged, with a shorter 'trouble-shooting' course being used before returning to intensive topical regimes.

How can I help with research into eczema?

If you would like to help from a financial viewpoint, there are a number of charities and skin research funds that provide money for scientists and dermatologists to embark on research projects into eczema. The best way to find out about these is to contact the National Eczema Society or the British Association of Dermatologists (see Appendix 1). We should also mention that these two groups are involved with the All Party Parliamentary Group on Skin (contact details in Appendix 1). This group is very useful as it helps to inform Parliament about the amount of skin disease in the UK and the impact it has on individuals and their families. It acts as a useful lobbying group when it comes to allocating medical resources for research care and training.

If you are interested in finding out about new trials in eczema treatment, again the National Eczema Society and the British Association of Dermatologists will give you up-to-date information about these and, if you are interested, how you can take part.

Glossary

Terms in *italic* in the definitions below are also defined in this Glossary.

acute Short-lasting. In medical terms, this usually means lasting for days rather than weeks or months. (*See also* chronic)

adrenal glands Important glands in the body that produce a number of *hormones* to control the body systems. Cortisol and cortisone are two very important examples, and adrenaline is another.

allergens If you are allergic to something, allergens are the tiny particles or substances to which you react when you come into contact with them.

allergy To have an allergy means to overreact to something in a harmful way when you come into contact with it. If you have an allergy to grass pollen, you will have streaming eyes and nose and sneezing if you come into contact with it (hayfever). Someone who is not allergic to grass pollen will not even notice when they have come into contact with it.

anaemia This means a reduction in the amount of the oxygen-carrying pigment, haemoglobin, in the blood.

anaphylaxis An abnormal reaction to a particular *antigen*, which can lead to breathing problems, a skin rash, swelling and collapse.

androgens These are *hormones* that stimulate the development of male sex organs and male secondary sexual characteristics (e.g. beard growth, deepening of the voice and muscle development). Very low levels are found in females.

anecdotal evidence Reports from people about their experience of *triggers*, treatments, etc. – rather than scientific evidence obtained from strictly regulated tests.

antibody A special kind of blood protein made in response to a particular *antigen*, which is designed to attack the antigen.

antigen Any substance that the body regards as foreign or potentially dangerous.

antihistamine A drug that inhibits the action of histamine, which is one of the substances in the body involved in producing allergic reactions.

atopic To be atopic is to have an inherited tendency to develop allergic or hypersensitive reactions. The three common atopic diseases are asthma, eczema and hay fever.

atrophy Wasting away of a body tissue. With skin, this means thinning and loss of strength.

barrier cream A cream or ointment used to protect the skin against irritants.

blister A swelling within the skin containing watery fluid, and sometimes blood or pus.

bone marrow The tissue contained in the internal cavities of bones that is involved in making blood cells.

chronic In strictly medical terms, chronic means long-lasting or persistent. Many people use the word 'chronic' incorrectly to mean severe or extreme. (*See also* acute)

dermatitis Another word for eczema, often used to imply that the cause is external rather than from within the body.

dermatology The medical speciality concerned with the diagnosis and treatment of skin disease.

dermis The deep layer of the skin.

diagnostic Something that is 'diagnostic' is a characteristic feature; it occurs so often in a disease that you do not need any other clues to know what the disease is.

distribution The pattern of a disease on the skin, for example all over, on the hands, in the *flexures*, etc.

eczema A red, itchy inflammation of the skin, sometimes with blisters and weeping.

ELISA This stands for enzyme-linked immunosorbent assay; it is a sensitive technique to measure the amount of a substance in the blood by using *antibodies.*

emollient An agent that soothes and softens the skin; also known as a moisturiser.

emulsifying ointment A thick, greasy *emollient.*

epidermis The outer layer of the skin.

erythroderma An abnormal reddening, flaking and thickening of the skin, affecting a wide area of the body.

extensor The side of a limb on which lie the muscles that straighten the limb (e.g. the back of the arm and the front of the leg).

flexures The areas where the limbs bend, bringing two skin surfaces close together (e.g. the creases at the front of the elbows, the back of the knees and the groin).

folliculitis An inflammation of the *hair follicles* in the skin.

genes 'Units' of inheritance that make up an individual's characteristics. Half are inherited from each parent.

genetic To do with *genes*.

hair follicles A specialised group of cells in the *dermis* that surround the root of a hair.

health visitor A trained nurse with experience in midwifery and special training in preventive medicine and education. Most health visitors deal with young children, but some specialise in care of the elderly.

herpes virus One of the agents that can produce infections that can lie dormant in the body. Examples are herpes simplex causing cold sores, and herpes zoster causing chickenpox and shingles.

hormone A substance that is produced in a gland in one part of the body and is carried in the bloodstream to work in other parts of the body.

house dust mite A microscopic insect that survives by feeding on the dead scales of human skin that make up house dust.

IgE Immunoglobulin E – one of a group of special proteins that act as *antibodies*.

immune system The body's defence system against outside 'attackers', whether they are infections, injuries or agents that are recognised as 'foreign' (e.g. a transplanted organ). The immune system fights off infection and produces *antibodies* that will protect against future attack.

immunity Resistance to specific disease(s) because of *antibodies* produced by the body's *immune system*.

immunosuppressive A drug that reduces the body's resistance to infection and other foreign bodies by suppressing the immune reaction.

inpatient therapy Treatment carried out when a patient is admitted to hospital.

incidence The number of new cases of an illness arising in a population over a given time.

inflammation The reaction of the body to an injury, infection or disease. It will generally protect the body against the spread of injury or infection, but it may become *chronic*, when it tends to damage the body rather than protect it.

interleukin-2 One of a group of special proteins that control the immune response. Interleukin-2 stimulates the T-*lymphocytes* that are active in the skin.

keratinocytes Types of cells that make up over 95% of the *epidermis* (outer layer of the skin).

lichenification Thickening of the *epidermis*, with exaggeration of the normal skin creases. The cause is excessive scratching or rubbing of the skin.

lymphocytes White blood cells that are involved in *immunity*.

malnutrition The condition resulting from an improper balance between what is eaten and what the body needs.

moisturiser *See* emollient.

natural history The normal course of a disease; the way it develops over time.

neurotransmitters Chemicals in the brain and nervous system that relay electrical messages between nerve cells.

paediatrician A doctor who is a specialist in diseases of childhood.

papular A pattern of rash that consists of small raised spots on the skin that are less than 5 mm across.

patch test A test to discover which *allergen* is responsible for contact *dermatitis*.

pH The number reflects how acidic or alkaline a substance is: 7 is neutral,; a lower figure indicates acidic; a higher figure indicates alkaline.

phototherapy Treatment with light – usually ultraviolet (UV) light.

placebo A medicine that is ineffective but may help to relieve a condition because the patient has faith in its powers. New drugs are tested against placebos to make sure that they have a true active benefit in addition to the 'placebo response'.

pompholyx A type of eczema on the hands and feet. Because the skin is so thick, the tiny *blisters* do not rupture, so they persist in the skin – causing intense itching.

psoriasis A *chronic* inflammatory skin disease, which can sometimes appear very similar to eczema.

psychologist A specialist who studies behaviour and its related mental processes.

pustule A small pus-containing *blister*.

sebaceous glands Glands in the skin that produce an oily substance – sebum.

seborrhoeic Related to excessive secretion of sebum. (*See also* sebaceous glands)

seborrhoeic eczema A form of eczema that affects the face, scalp, upper back and chest. It characteristically produces yellowish, greasy scales.

steroids A particular group of chemicals, which includes very important *hormones*, produced naturally by the body, as well as many drugs used for a wide range of medical purposes. In eczema, the subgroup of steroids with which we are concerned is the corticosteroids. This term is very often shortened to 'steroids', causing people to confuse their skin treatments with the anabolic steroids used for body-building.

subcutaneous Beneath the skin.

systemic This term is used for a drug, given by mouth or injection, that affects the whole body.

topical A term used to describe drugs that are applied to the skin rather than being taken internally.

triggers Factors that may bring on eczema but do not cause eczema.

urticaria An itchy rash, looking like a nettle sting, caused by the release of histamine (*see also* antihistamine). Swellings on the skin appear rapidly and disappear within hours.

Appendix 1
Useful addresses

Please note that website addresses change quite frequently and quickly become out of date.

Patient support organisations

National Eczema Society
Hill House
Highgate Hill
London N19 5NA
Tel: 020 7281 3553
Fax: 020 7281 6395
Eczema Information Line:
0870 241 3604
(Mon–Fri 8 am – 8 pm)
Email: helpline@eczema.org
Website: www.eczema.org
An organisation dedicated to meeting the needs of people with eczema and their families, providing advice, support and information, including lists of cotton stockists and specialist bedding manufacturers, and encouraging research.

Changing Faces
1 & 2 Junction Mews
London W2 1PN
Tel: 0845 4500275
Email: info@changingfaces.co.uk
Website: www.changingfaces.co.uk
A charity that helps people facially disfigured in any way to express themselves with more confidence, and combats many of their anxieties and negative feelings.

Skin Care Campaign
Hill House
Highgate Hill
London N19 5NA
Tel: 020 7561 8248
Website: www.skincarecampaign.org
An alliance of patient groups, health professionals and other organisations concerned with skin care. It campaigns for a better deal for people with a wide variety of skin problems.

Skinship
Plascow Cottage
Kirkgunzeon
Dumfries DG2 8JT
Tel: 01387 760567
*Provides a helpline for people
with any skin disease.*

Government websites and guidelines

Action on Dermatology
www.modern.nhs.uk/action-on

Benefit Enquiry Line
Room 901
Victoria House
Ormskirk Road
Preston
Lancashire PR1 2QP
Tel: 0800 88 22 00
Fax: 01772 238953
Website: www.dwp.gov.uk
*State benefits information line
for sick or disabled people and
their carers.*

**Department for Education
and Skills**
www.dfes.gov.uk

Department of Health
www.doh.gov.uk

**Department of Work
and Pensions**
www.dwp.gov.uk
Go to
www.dwp.gov.uk/localoffice/disability
for addresses of Disability
Benefits Centres.

Directgov
www.direct.gov.uk
*For up-to-date government and
public service information.*

Health & Safety Executive
www.hse.gov.uk

**National Electronic Library
for Health (NeLH)**
www.nelh.nhs.uk
and then go through to Specialist
Libraries – SKIN.
*Provides health-care
professionals and the public
(through NHS Direct Online and
the New Library Network) with
knowledge and know-how to
support health-care-related
decisions.*

**National Institute for Health
and Clinical Excellence**
www.nice.org.uk
*Gives guidance on the use
of treatments and disease
management strategies.
Can also be accessed through
the National Electronic Library
for Health (above).*

National Research Register (NRR)
www.nrr.nhs.uk
A database of ongoing and recently completed research projects funded by, or of interest to, the UK's National Health Service.

Other useful sources of information

All Party Parliamentary Group on Skin
26 Cadogan Street
London SW1X 0JP
Tel: 020 7591 4833
Fax: 020 7591 4831
An all-party group specialising in skin, which was established in 1993 to raise awareness in Parliament of skin disease.

Association of the British Pharmaceutical Industry
12 Whitehall
London SW1A 2DY
Tel: 020 7930 3477
Fax: 020 7747 1411
Email: abpi@abpi.org.uk
Brings together companies in Britain that produce prescription medicines, other organisations involved in pharmaceutical research and development, and those with an interest in the pharmaceutical industry in the UK.

Asthma UK
Summit House
70 Wilson Street
London EC2A 2DB
Tel: 020 7786 4900
Email: info@asthma.org.uk
Website: www.asthma.org.uk

British Association of Dermatologists (BAD) / British Dermatological Nursing Group (BDNG)
4 Fitzroy Square
London W1T 5HQ
Tel: 020 7383 0266
Fax: 020 7388 5263
Email: admin@bad.org.uk
Websites: www.bad.org.uk
www.bdng.org.uk
Professional organisations representing doctors and nurses who have an interest in and/or work directly in dermatology. Among other things, the organisations provide patient information leaflets about various skin diseases, including eczema.

**British Association
of Skin Camouflage**
PO Box 202
Macclesfield
Cheshire SK11 6FP
Tel: 01625 871129
Email: info@skin-camouflage.net
Website: www.skin-camouflage.net
*A network of practitioners
trained in camouflage
techniques for skin conditions
and disfiguring injuries.*

**British Homeopathic
Association**
29 Park Street West
Luton
Bedfordshire LU1 3BE
Tel: 0870 4443950
Website: trusthomeopathy.org
*To promote homeopathy and
encourage its understanding
and use by the public while
campaigning for more
homeopathy on the NHS.*

**British Medical
Acupuncture Society**
BMAS House
3 Winnington Court
Northwich
Cheshire CW8 1AQ
Tel: 01606 786782
Fax: 01606 786783
Email:
admin@medical-acupuncture.org.uk
Website:
www.medical-acupuncture.co.uk

British Red Cross Society
44 Moorfields
London EC2Y 9AL
Tel: 0870 170 7000
Website: www.redcross.org.uk
*Offers a camouflage service
using special techniques to cover
up unwanted skin changes.*

Citizens Advice Bureau
Website: www.nacab.org.uk
*For a wide range of advice,
including financial and state
benefits. Look in the telephone
directory for your local branch.*

**Institute for
Complementary Medicine**
PO Box 194
London SE16 7QZ
Tel: 020 7237 5165
(weekdays 10 am – 2 pm)
Fax: 020 7237 5175
Website: www.i-c-m.org.uk
*Information and advice about
complementary therapy.*

**Long-Term Medical
Conditions Alliance**
Unit 212
16 Baldwins Gardens
London EC1N 7RJ
Tel: 020 7813 3637
Fax: 020 7813 3640
Email: info@lmca.org.uk
Website: www.lmca.org.uk
*Made up of over 100
organisations, the Alliance
campaigns on behalf of people*

with long-term medical conditions.

Motability Operations
City Gate House
22 Southwark Bridge Road
London SE1 9HB
Tel: 0845 456 4566
Fax: 020 7928 1818
Website: www.motability.co.uk
Advice and help about cars, scooters and wheelchairs for people with disabilities.

NHS Direct
0845 4647
A 24-hour helpline, manned by nurses, for information about health.

Primary Care Dermatology Society
Gable House
40 High Street
Rickmansworth
Hertfordshire WD3 1ER
Tel: 01923 711678
Email: pcds@pcds.org.uk
Website: www.pcds.org.uk
An organisation made up of GPs who have a special interest in dermatology.

Royal College of Nursing (RCN)
20 Cavendish Square
London W1G 0RN
Tel: 020 7409 3333
Website: www.rcn.org.uk

Skin Treatment and Research Trust (START)
Chelsea and Westminster
Hospital
369 Fulham Road
London SW10 9NH
Tel: 020 8746 8174
Primarily a laboratory research establishment rather than an information service, but they may be able to give information about specific research questions.

Society of Homeopaths
11 Brookfield
Duncan Close
Moulton Park
Norhampton NN3 6WL
Tel: 0845 450 6611
Fax: 0845 450 6622
Email: info@homeopathy-soh.org
Website: www.homeopathy-soh.com
A professional organisation for homeopaths, but it offers a service of finding a homeopath in your area.

Informative websites

www.bnf.org
Gives sound, up-to-date information on the use of medicines

www.bsid.org.uk
Promotes research in dermatology

www.bupa.co.uk/health_information
Fact sheets that can be downloaded

www.dermatlas.org
A site with many different images of skin disease

www.dermatology.co.uk
An independent website providing an educational resource on skin conditions and their treatment to patients, the public and health professionals

www.dermnetnz.org
Award-winning website of the New Zealand Dermatological Society; aims to provide authoritative information about the skin for health professionals and patients with skin diseases

www.DermQuest.com
Another site with many images of skin disease

www.familyfund.org.uk
For information on the Family Fund

www.fihealth.org.uk
The Prince of Wales Foundation for Integrated Health

www.google.com
Then enter "disease + emedicine" for the search

www.gpnotebook.co.uk
Oxbridge Solutions is an encyclopaedia of medical information for GPs

www.ifd.org
The International Foundation for Dermatology

www.mhra.gov.uk
The Medicines and Healthcare products Regulatory Agency

www.patient.co.uk
A patient UK medical search engine

www.sign.ac.uk
The Scottish Intercollegiate Guidelines Network, which gives unbiased guidance on best medical practice through a systematic evaluation of clinical evidence

www.which.net/health/dtb
Website for the Drug & Therapeutics Bulletin, which provides advice on treatments and patient notes

Appendix 2
Useful publications

Special Educational Needs – A Guide for Parents and Carers, Department of Education and Employment.

Traveller's Guide to Health, Department of Health. Contact the Department of Health on 0845 606 2030, or go to www.doh.gov.uk.

The National Eczema Society (contact details in Appendix 1) provide a wide range of written information on all aspects of eczema.

Index

The *'At Your Fingertips'* guide Feedback Form

We hope that you found *Eczema – the 'at your fingertips' guide* helpful. We always appreciate readers' opinions and would be grateful if you could take a few minutes to complete this form for us.

❶ How did you acquire your copy of this book?

From my local library ☐

Read an article in a newspaper/magazine ☐

Found it by chance ☐

Recommended by a friend ☐

Recommended by a patient organisation/charity ☐

Recommended by a doctor/nurse/advisor ☐

Saw an advertisement ☐

❷ How much of the book have you read?

All of it ☐

More than half of it ☐

Less than half of it ☐

❸ Which copies/chapters have been most helpful?

....

....

❹ Overall, how useful to you was this *'at your fingertips'* guide?

Extremely useful ☐

Very useful ☐

Useful ☐

❺ What did you find most helpful?

....

....

6 **What did you find least helpful?**

....

....

7 **Have you read any other health books?**

       Yes ☐   No ☐

If yes, which subjects did they cover?

....

....

How did this '*at your fingertips*' guide compare?

Much better   ☐

Better   ☐

About the same   ☐

Not as good   ☐

8 **Would you recommend this book to a friend?**

       Yes ☐   No ☐

Thank you for your help. Please send your completed form to:

Class Publishing, FREEPOST, London W6 7BR

Surname   First name

Title Prof/Dr/Mr/Mrs/Ms

Address

Town   Postcode   Country

☐ Please add my name and address to receive details of related books

    [Please note, we will not pass on your details to any other company]

Have you found **Eczema – the 'at your fingertips' guide** useful and practical? If so, you may be interested in other books from Class Publishing.

Acne
– the 'at your fingertips' guide   £17.99
Dr Tim Mitchell and Alison Dudley
Acne is the most common chronic skin condition of adolescents, affecting to some extent almost all teenage boys and girls. It tends to begin at puberty, and while for most people it tends to go away by the time they reach their mid-20s, some people may continue to have acne until they reach their 40s or 50s.
'By far the best book I have read on the subject.' – *Peter Lapsley, Chief Executive, Skin Care Campaign*

Asthma
– the 'at your fingertips' guide   £17.99
Dr Mark Levy, Trisha Weller and Professor Sean Hilton
Asthma – the 'at your fingertips' guide contains over 250 real questions from people with asthma and their families – answered by three medical experts. This handbook contains up-to-date, medically accurate and practical advice on living with asthma.
'A unique resource for those with asthma.' – *Dr Martyn Partridge, Chief Medical Adviser, National Asthma Campaign*

Heart Health
– the 'at your fingertips' guide   £14.99
Dr Graham Jackson
This practical handbook, written by a leading cardiologist, answers all your questions about heart conditions. It tells you all about you and your heart; how to keep your heart healthy, or if it has been affected by heart disease – how to make it as strong as possible.
'Those readers who want to know more about the various treatments for heart disease will be much enlightened.' – *Dr James Le Fanu, Daily Telegraph*

Kidney Dialysis and Transplants
– the 'at your fingertips' guide   £14.99
Dr Andy Stein and Janet Wild with Juliet Auer
A practical handbook for anyone with long-term kidney failure or their families. The book contains answers to over 450 real questions actually asked by people with end-stage renal failure, and offers positive, clear and medically accurate advice on every aspect of living with the condition.
'A first class book on kidney dialysis and transplants that is simple and accurate, and can be used to equal advantage by doctors and their patients.' – *Dr Thomas Stuttaford, The Times*

Diabetes
– the 'at your fingertips' guide   £14.99
Professor Peter Sönksen, Dr Charles Fox and Sue Judd
This is an invaluable reference guide for people with diabetes, which offers practical advice on every aspect of living with the condition, giving you the knowledge and reassurance you need to deal confidently with your diabetes.
'I have no hesitation in commending this book.' – *Sir Steve Redgrave CBE, Vice President, Diabetes UK*

High Blood Pressure
– the 'at your fingertips' guide   £14.99
Dr Tom Fahey, Professor Deirdre Murphy with Dr Julian Tudor Hart
The authors use all their years of experience as blood pressure experts to answer your questions on high blood pressure, in order to give you the information you need to bring your blood pressure down – and keep it down.
'Readable and comprehensive information' – *Dr Sylvia McLaughlan, Director General, The Stroke Association*

PRIORITY ORDER FORM

Cut out or photocopy this form and send it (post free in the UK) to:
Class Publishing
FREEPOST 16705
Macmillan Distribution
Basingstoke   **Tel: 01256 302 699**
RG21 6ZZ   **Fax: 01256 812 558**

Please send me urgently   *Post included*
(tick boxes below)   *price per copy (UK only)*

☐ **Eczema – the 'at your fingertips' guide**   £17.99
   (ISBN 10: 1859591256 / ISBN 13: 9781859591253)

☐ **Acne – the 'at your fingertips' guide**   £20.99
   (ISBN 10: 185959073X / ISBN 13: 9781859590737)

☐ **Asthma – the 'at your fingertips' guide**   £20.99
   (ISBN 10: 1859591116 /ISBN 13: 9781859591116)

☐ **Heart Health – the 'at your fingertips' guide**   £17.99
   (ISBN 10: 1859590977 / ISBN 13: 9781859590973)

☐ **Diabetes – the 'at your fingertips' guide**   £17.99
   (ISBN 10: 185959087X / ISBN 13: 9781859590874)

☐ **High Blood Pressure – the 'at your fingertips' guide**   £17.99
   (ISBN 10: 185959090X / ISBN 13: 9781859590904)

☐ **Kidney Dialysis and Transplants – the 'at your fingertips' guide**   £17.99
   (ISBN 10: 1859590462 / ISBN 13: 9781859590641)

                                                     TOTAL _____

Easy ways to pay

Cheque: I enclose a cheque payable to Class Publishing for £ _____

Credit card: Please debit my   ☐ Mastercard   ☐ Visa   ☐ Amex

Number _____ Expiry date _____

Name _____

My address for delivery is _____

Town _____ County _____ Postcode _____

Telephone number *(in case of query)* _____

Credit card billing address if different from above _____

Town _____ County _____ Postcode _____

Class Publishing's guarantee: remember that if, for any reason, you are not satisfied with these books, we will refund all your money, without any questions asked. Prices and VAT rates may be altered for reasons beyond our control.